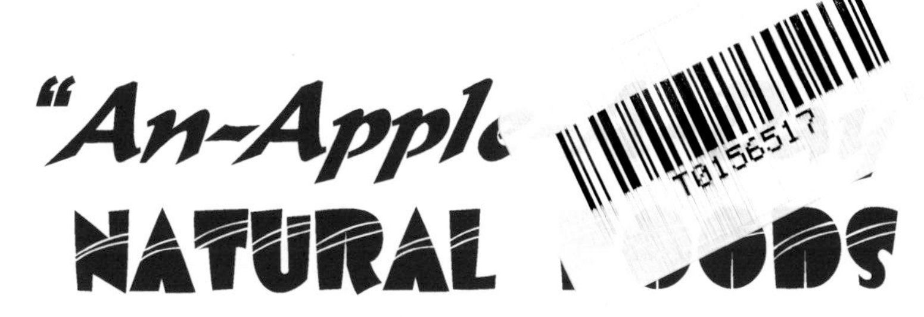


and their nutritional value

# FOR
# A HEALTHIER AND YOUNGER YOU

George Edward Weigel

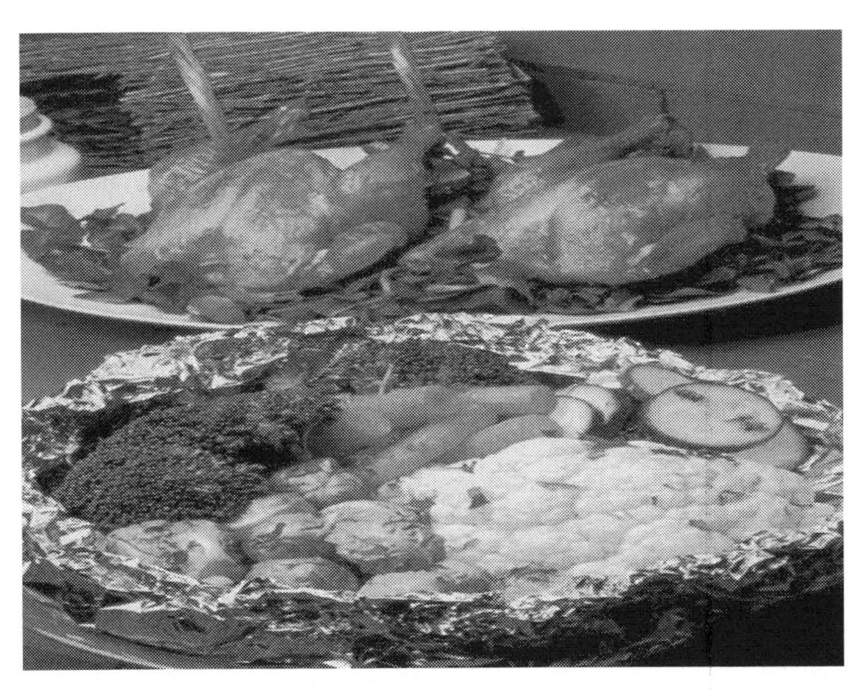

"An-Apple-A-Day"
Natural Foods



You should not undertake any diet/exercise regimen recommended in this book before consulting your personal physician. Neither the author nor the publisher shall be responsible or liable for any loss or damage allegedly arising as a consequence of your use or application of any information or suggestions contained in this book.

iUniverse books may be ordered through booksellers or by contacting:

iUniverse
1663 Liberty Drive
Bloomington, IN 47403
www.iuniverse.com
1-800-Authors (1-800-288-4677)



ISBN: 978-1-4502-1500-8 (pbk)
ISBN: 978-1-4502-1501-5 (ebk)

Printed in the United States of America

iUniverse rev. date: 4/09/2010

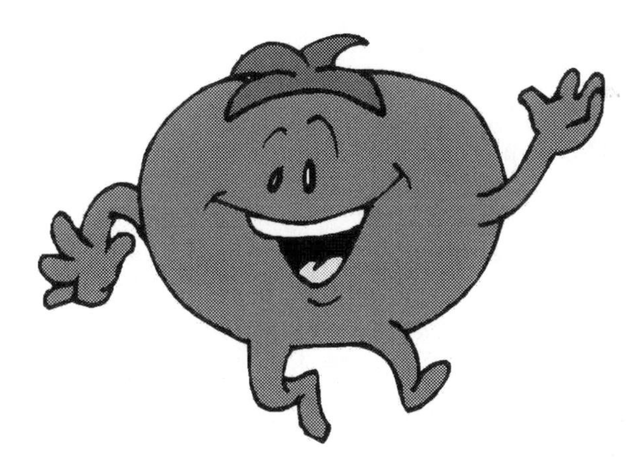

**The first step to turning your life and health around was picking up this book!**

# Nutrition the apple

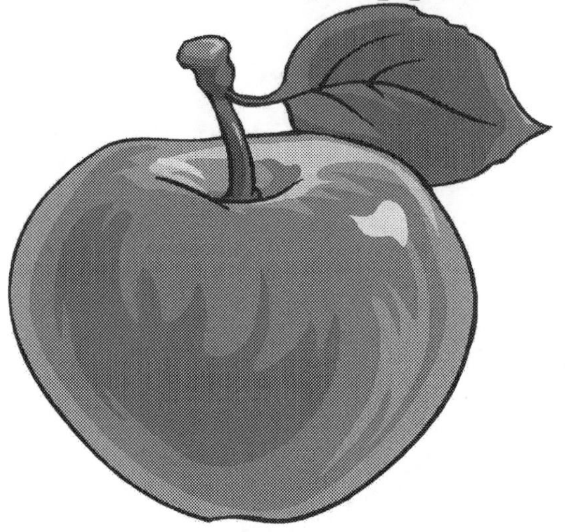

You have heard, ***"An-Apple-A-Day will keep the doctor away."*** While it will certainly take more than a daily apple to keep you healthy, it is a step in the right direction. Apples are delicious, easy to carry for snacking, low in calories, a natural mouth freshener, and they are still very inexpensive.

Apples are a source of both soluble and insoluble fiber. Soluble fiber such as pectin actually helps to prevent cholesterol buildup in the lining of blood vessel walls, thus reducing the incident of atherosclerosis and heart disease. The soluble fiber in apples provides bulk in the intestinal tract, holding water to cleanse and move food quickly through the digestive system.

It is a good idea to eat apples with their skin. Almost half of the vitamin C content is just underneath the skin. Eating the skin also increases insoluble fiber content. Most of an apple's fragrance cells are also concentrated in the skin and they ripen, the skin cells develop more aroma and flavor.

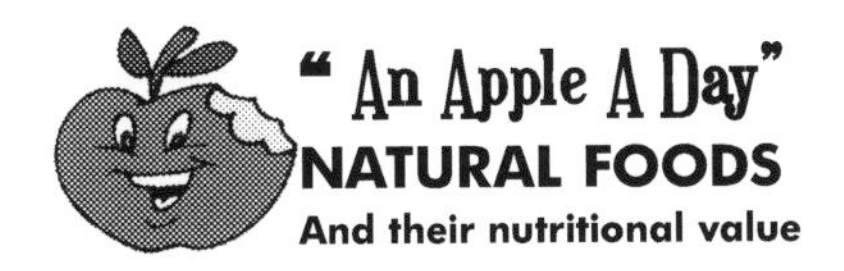


AUTHOR: George Edward Weigel

Graphics & design: George Edward Weigel

Publisher: iuniverse

Research by: Cedar Creek Research (A George Edward Weigel Enterprise)

**Printed and bound in the USA**



NOTE: The information in this book is not intended as a substitute for medical treatment and advice. It is advisable to consult a medical professional before using any of these methods. Particularly if you or suffering from a medical condition and are unsure of the suitability of any of the remedies of foods mentioned in this book. A dietitian or doctor should be consulted before any change in diet.

"An-Apple-A-Day"

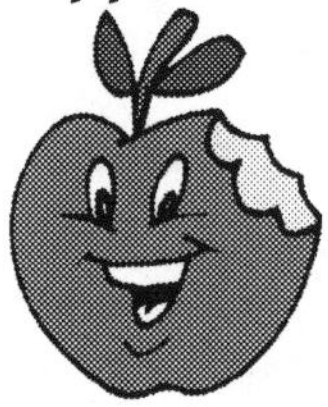

Mother earth has bless us with an abundance
of natural nutritional organically delicious foods,
for our health and well-being!

# CONTENTS

**“an-apple-a-day”**
**“keeps-the-the-doctor-away”**

You may be eating plenty of food, but not eating the right foods that will give your body the nutrients you need to be healthy.

“Your body has trillions of cells, each one demanding a constant supply of daily nutrients, which you will get from eating natural nutritional foods, which will keep your body functioning.

Eating these natural foods is the key to a healthy lifestyle, and helps balanced brain function, and energy.

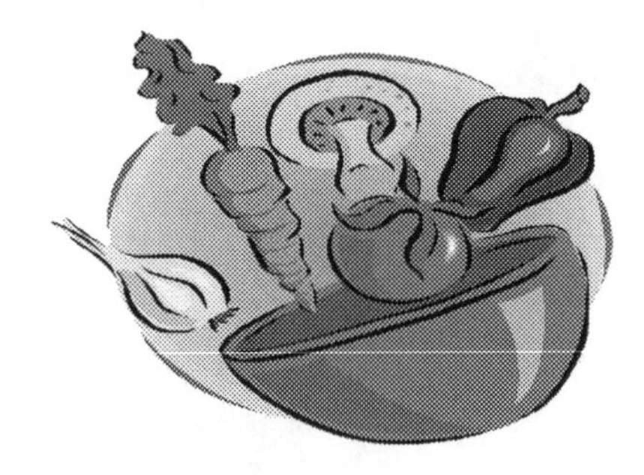

# Introduction:

## Why are fruit, vegetables and whole grains so amazingly good for you?

Here in this Book you will find, easy-to-understand information about the essential nutrients packed into these natural foods. Read the importance of natural healthy foods such as fruit, vegetables, grains and nuts. Also this book will give all the information you need to make informed decisions about your health and nutritional safety.

Good natural healthy food is the basis of good health. We must make healthy conscious food choices for maximum health benefits. Fresh fruits and vegetables, whole grains, nuts and legumes – all of these must be a part of our everyday diet. They are rich in the photochemical that fight diseases like osteoporosis, cancer and heart disease.

Natural healthy foods also called whole foods are those which are grown and prepared in a more natural way than most commercially processed foods. Natural foods includes organic food, functional food and food for particular nutritional uses. These type of foods are becoming popular because, they are considered to be better than commercially produced foods. It is essential to ensure an adequate intake of natural nutritional healthy foods on a daily basis.

Healthy foods can be categorized into five main categories. The first includes stone-ground, whole wheat breads, cereals and flavours. The second category comprises cold pressed, unrefined oils and unsalted nuts. The third category of natural foods are yogurt and low-fat milk made without preservatives. The fourth is free-range eggs, those not laid by production hens. The Fifth category of natural food includes fruit and vegetables grown in soil fed with organic matter such as farmyard manure, leaves, grass clippings etc.

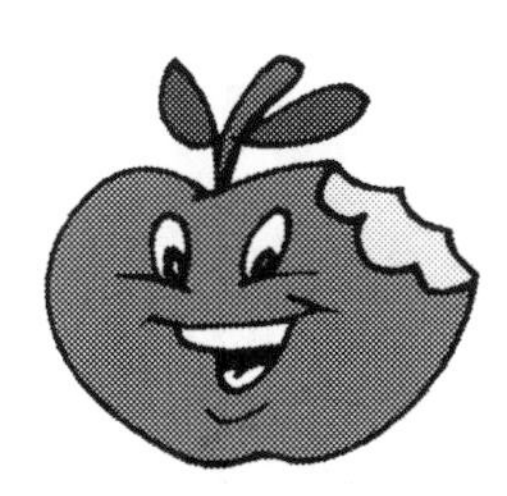

# CHAPTER 1

# Types of natural Nutritional Food

# Types of Natural Nutritional Foods, from mother earth to your table!

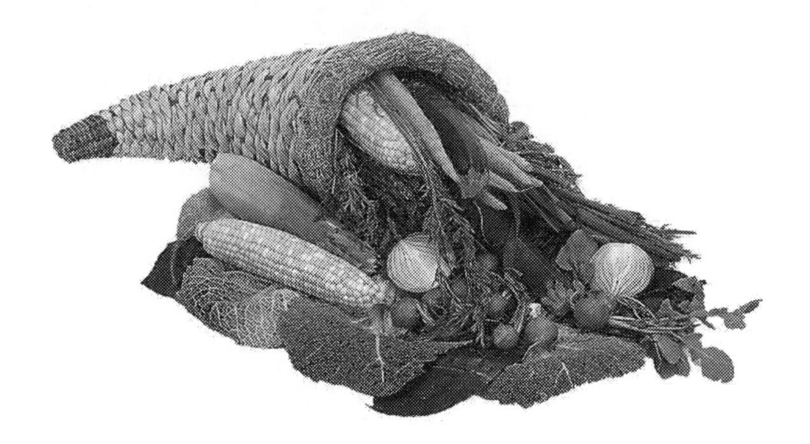

A diet in nutrients and low in additives and preservatives is the key to great health. If you truly start to eat all of these different natural foods. I can assure you that you will be doing a great service to your body's general overall health. If you adopt this diet, you will feel stronger, sexier, more energized and happier. It is essential to ensure an adequate intake of natural healthy foods on a daily basis. Adding variety by changing the foods we eat or experimenting with new flavors ensures we stick to eating healthy. However, this does not mean totally cutting out on foods we enjoy, like barbecue, cake, etc. These should be occasional treats. And will help you stay on your healthy diet. In a nutshell discover and explorer the many mouthwatering healthy foods waiting to tantalize your taste buds. Eating a balanced nutrient-rich diet will help you break this cycle of cravings, sugar and weight gain. This is because eating well not only nourishes your body but regulates your blood sugar levels so that you don't get those lows when you crave sugar pick-me-ups. Your energy levels are less likely to dip, which means you are less likely to crave food that you don't need or is not good for you.

## Natural Nutritional Food List:

Organic food, functional food and food for particular nutritional uses are considered to be better than commercially produced food.

| Vegetables | Leafy green vegetables | Grains |
|---|---|---|
| Artichoke | Beet greens | Amaranth |
| Asparagus | Chicory | Barley |
| Avocado | Collards | Basmati rice |
| Beets | Dandelion greens | Brown rice |
| Broccoli | Endive | Buckwheat |
| Brussels sprouts | Escarole | Bulgur wheat |
| Cabbage | Iceberg lettuce | Corn |
| Carrots | Kale | Kamut |
| Cauliflower | Loose-leaf-lettuce | Millet |
| Celeriac | Mache | Oats |
| Celery | Mustard greens | Quinoa |
| Eggplant | Turnip greens | Rye |
| Green peas | Parsley | Spelt |
| Okra | Rocket | Whole wheat |
| Onions | Romaine | |
| Parsley | Sorrel | |
| Parsnip | Spinach | |
| Peppers | Swiss chard | |
| Potato | Watercress | |
| Radish | | |
| Squash | | |
| Tomato | | |
| Turnip | | |
| Watercress | | |
| Yam | | |
| Zucchini | | |

| Fruit | Fruit | Nuts |
|---|---|---|
| Apples | Loganberries | Almonds |
| Apricots | Orange | Brazil nuts |
| Blackberries | Passion fruit | Cashews * |
| Blueberries | Pineapples | Filberts |
| Cherries | Pomegranates | Hazelnuts |
| Grapes | Strawberries | Chestnuts |
| Guavas | Tangelos | Pecans |
| Huckleberries | Tangerines | Pine nuts |
| Kiwi fruits | All dried fruit | Pistachios |
| Loquats | Bananas | Walnuts |
| Lychees | Dates | |
| Mangos | Figs | |
| Mulberries | Melons | |
| Nectarines | Cantaloupe | |
| Papayas | Honeydew | |
| Peaches | Watermelon | |
| Pears | | |
| Cactus fruit | | |
| Cranberries | | |
| Currants | | |
| Dates | | |
| Gooseberries | | |
| Grapefruit | | |
| Kumquat | | |
| Lemons | | |
| Limes | | |

* (in moderation)

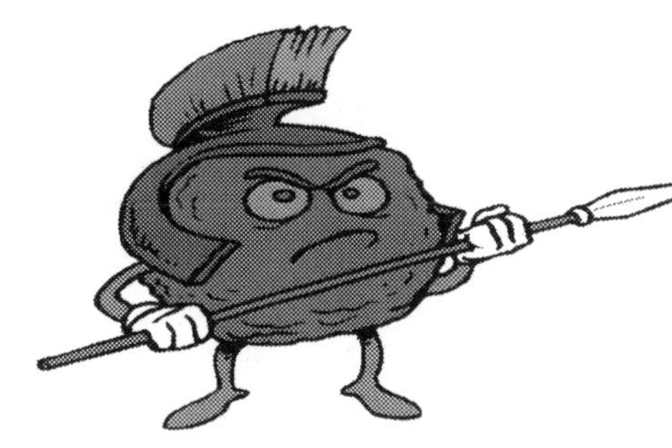

# Protect Your health By eating good natural foods

By combining fruits, vegetables, nuts, seeds, whole grains, lean meat, fish, free range eggs, dairy products, herbs and spices with plenty of water at lest seven to eight glasses a day. We achieve a diet full of life-enhancing nutrients. These give the body the necessary means to keep healthy and to function efficiently, which in turn helps us feel fitter and look younger. Studies continue to tell us that Americans fall shot of meeting the minimum nutritional requirements to stay healthy.

*Most people are falling way short of providing the nutritional needs to perform at our best both physically and mentally*

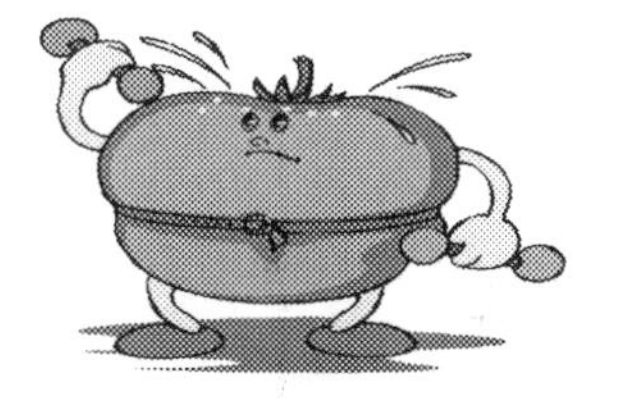

A healthy diet consists of plenty of fruits and vegetables and whole grains (preferably organic). Fruits and vegetables fresh; fresh frozen is still good but not as good as "off the farm fresh"! Recent studies indicate that a lot of people in the U.S. Are eating in restaurants rather than in the home. Restaurant food tends to be too high in fat, sugar, high processed foods, etc. Convenience foods now make up a much higher percentage of the average diet than in the past. In some people their food is from so-called "empty calorie foods (candy, sweets, chips,or other high processed foods that lack nutritional value other than calories. Remember that the more highly processed a food is, the more likely it is falling short of nutritional value. Also the greater the external stresses, the more nutritional demands on the body. Eating a poor quality diet robs you of nutritional factors necessary for good health.

There are good carbs, these are carbs without the added refined sugar. Fruits, whole grain breads, rice and many vegetables. These natural healthy carbohydrates (complex carbs) contain naturally occurring sugars that the body can slowly and easily metabolize. These help balanced brain function, and energy. Also there are good fats, such as foods like nuts, seeds, etc. these natural foods are oil-rich contain healthy fats which are necessary for aiding weight reduction, lowering cholesterol, your immunity and nourishing the skin, hair, bone and lubricating the body. They are so important that they are called essential fatty acids (EFAs). Your body cannot make EFAs, so you must get them from the foods you eat. These are good fats and necessary for life itself. Also lets not forget protein, vegetable proteins are easy to break down in the body. And are a more efficient, healthier and a lot cheaper form of protein than meat. When you combined beans and grains together they form a complete protein, easy to digest and metabolize. If you want the best natural foods than try organic foods. Organic means foods that are free of chemicals. Foods that are organic have been grown in soils that have no chemical fertilizers and pesticides. If chemicals have been used on the produce that you eat. Then those chemicals, which are toxic, will enter your body cells and bloodstream and could cause damage. There are numerous studies and research showing that chemicals entering our bodies do not help our health. Don't confuse natural foods with organic foods. The (USDA) defines "organic" food as food grown and processed without using most conventional pesticides, without fertilizers made with synthetic ingredients, without biotechnology, without ionizing radiation and without sewage sludge. I myself grow my own self- sustaining organic garden, raising my food for health, nutrition and cost. One of the delights of gardening is fresh vegetables and fruit. I also make my own organic compost, and homemade natural fertilizers and pesticides. You can read my other book **"The Blue Barn"** on self-sustaining organic gardening. If you have an interest in growing your own garden. It will get you off to a great start.

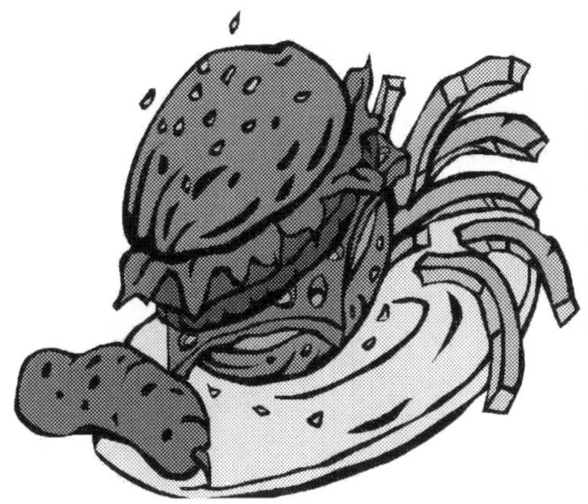

Basically if your diet isn't healthy, you won't feel healthy nor will you have the energy to enjoy a great full life. Many people are simply unaware of how to eat healthy. Taste and Convenience become the major part of their selection, while nutritional value is given little attention, if any at all. Many nutritional researchers point to the rising problems of obesity, diabetes and heart conditions as evidence of the quality of the diet most people consume. Unhealthy foods will accelerate the aging process, cause digestive problems, increase the pain and swelling of arthritis, give unhealthy-looking skin, hair and nails, weaken your immunity, give you mood swings, make arteries narrow and stiff which help the formation of blood clots, promote toxic activity within your body which years later could cause cancerous growth, increases the risk of heart disease and arthritis. Too many fatty foods, including red meats, dairy products, fried and junk foods, can clog the arteries, deplete calcium levels and excessive intake can cause heart problems and other vital organs. Also to much alcohol puts a strain on your digestive system and liver.

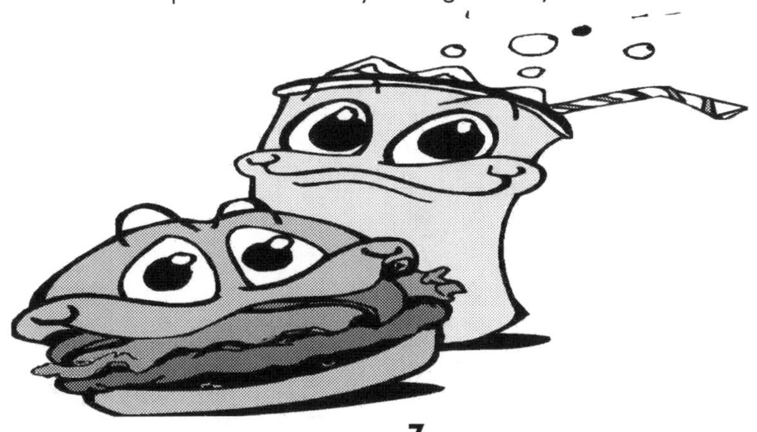

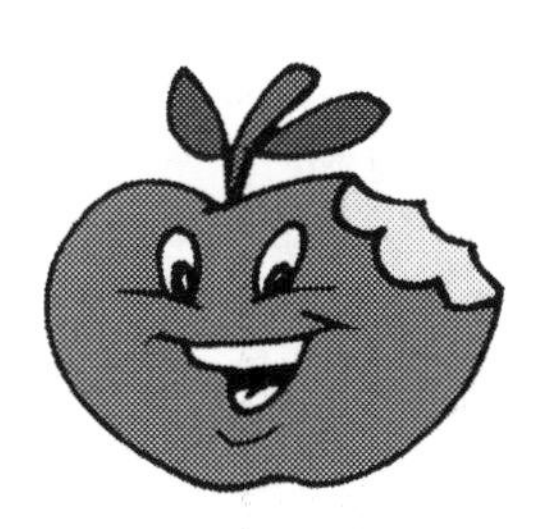

CHAPTER 2

# Healthy Natural Food Shopping

# Healthy "Natural" food shopping

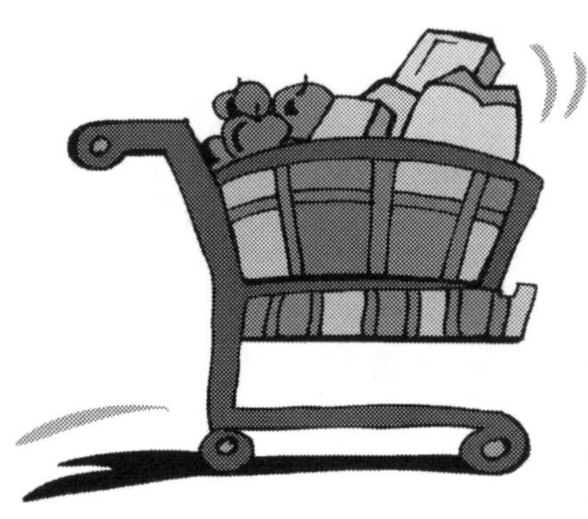

Healthy food shopping is an important part of making healthy meals, because what we buy at the food store or supermarket determines our food intake. Food shopping requires some planning beforehand. Following a few simple guidelines will help you make the most of your food shopping. Fruits and vegetables must be at the very top of the healthy food shopping list. A diet high in nutrients and low in additives and preservatives is the key to great health, but supermarkets can be confusing places with so many different types of foods. Use the following as a guide to help you choose which foods to include and which to avoid to maintain good health. When you walk through the supermarket, aim for the produce aisles first. This is an aisle bursting with energy from the raw, unadulterated fruit and vegetables, the way nature intended. Buy those in season to save money. Dark colored vegetables and fruits, for example, dark green and orange, are rich in vitamins and other nutrients your body needs for good health. Seek out those fruits and vegetables that seem to be the healthiest, that look in the best condition. Do not buy or eat old, decrepit looking, wilted fruits or vegetables. They will have no or very little nutrient content. Buy different varieties of wholegrain breads, low-sugar cereals and/or wholegrain, different pasta varieties wholegrain, brown rice and biscuits made of wholegrain flour and dried fruits. Buy alternatives to cream, mayonnaise, prepared sauces and high-fat salad dressing. Buy a variety of seasonings like black pepper, garlic, ginger and onion, spices and herbs (fresh and dried) Add some variety and spice to your everyday meals by experimenting with new flavors.

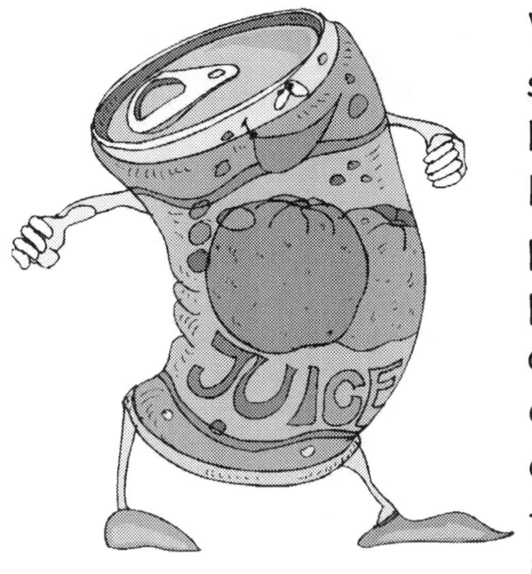


While food shopping choose healthy snacks for kids, like nuts, popcorn (air-popped), yogurt and avoid sugary drinks and aerated drinks. Choose fresh fruit juices instead.

Beverages including soda and soft drinks contain "empty calories" which are useless and they don't contain vitamins or minerals. There is also high content of carbon dioxide in these beverages.

There are good sweets, not all sweets are bad for you. A matter of fact, mother nature has provided us with an abundance of natural sweets we get them from our gardens and orchards and they are great for us. These are fruits given to us from the earth. Fruits are nutrient-rich and a good source of live enzymes and antioxidants to booster your immune system and energy levels. Here is a list of some of the best fruits, blueberries, blackberries, raspberries, strawberries, watermelon, apples, apricots, cherries, grapes, peaches, pears, plums. I would recommend you eat at least one of these fresh fruits a day, two would be better. Once again I grow all of these fruits in my orchard, and if you never had fresh ripened fruit right off the tree. Well you are missing a great delightful experience. Since sugars contribute calories with few, if any, nutrients, look for foods and beverages low in added sugar.

**NOTE:** It's always good to choose food that is organically produced as it has fewer chemicals and additives.

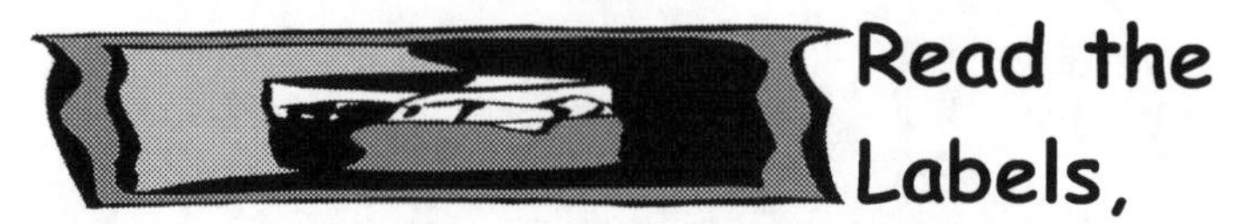

# Read the Labels, know the facts about nutrition

Most packaged foods have a nutrition facts label. For a healthier you, use this tool to make smart food choices quickly and easily. It's important to pay attention to food labels and get used to spotting hidden ingredients. Additives in our food have been linked to a variety of health problems including asthma, hyperactivity, headaches, allergies and even cancer. We are very fortunate today that food manufacturers are required to list the ingredients in products. Additives in the form of colorings, preservatives, emulsifies, flavor enhancers and thickeners these make the body's detox system less efficient and increase the toxic load.

**Try these tips:**

- Keep these additives low: saturated fats, trans fats, cholesterol, and sodium.
- Look for these: potassium, fiber, vitamins A and C, calcium, and iron.
- Use the % daily value (DV) column when possible, 5% DV or less is low, 20% DV or more is high.
- Check serving and calories, look at the serving size and how many servings you are actually consuming.
- Read the ingredient list and make sure that added sugars are not one of the first few ingredients. Some names for added sugars (caloric sweeteners) include sucrose, glucose, high fructose corn syrup, corn syrup, and fructose.
- Look for foods low in saturated fats, trans fats, and cholesterol, to help reduce the risk of heart disease 5% DV or less is low, 20% DV or more is high. Most of the fats you eat should be polyunsaturated and monounsaturated fats.

- Reduce sodium (salt), increase potassium. Research shows that eating less than 2,300 milligrams of sodium, about 1 tsp of salt per day my reduce the risk of high blood pressure. Most of the sodium people eat comes from processed foods, not the saltshaker. Also look for foods high in potassium, which counteracts some of sodium's effect on blood pressure.

## Here is a few more things to look for on labels

- **Thickeners, emulsifiers and stabilizers**, these are found in breads, cakes, cookies, margarine and other spreads, jams, sauces, soups, chocolate and milk shakes. Sodium is just another name for salt. Animal fat is saturated fat and trans-fatty acid is another name for hydrogenated fat. How can you tell when there is a long list of unknown chemical names. If that's the case, the general rule is to avoid the product
- **Preservatives,** the main function of preservatives is to extend a food's shelf life. Synthetic additives such as BHA and BHT (E320-21) may not be safe. They may promote the carcinogenic changes in cells caused by other substances. Alum, an aluminum compound, is used in many brands of pickles to increase crispiness. Aluminum has no place in the human body and you should avoid it. It is best to avoid products containing sodium nitrate or other nitrates, such as bacon, ham and hot dogs.
- **Colorings,** Stay clear of foods made with artificial colors. These are one of the easiest to avoid, the dyes capable of interacting with and damaging your immune system, speeding up aging, and may push you in the direction of cancer.

| Yea! | Nay! |
| --- | --- |
| **FRUIT:** Choose fresh, frozen or dried fruits without sweeteners, unsulfured fruits. Buy organic when possible. Fruit are high in essential vitamins, minerals, fiber and antioxidants. | Avoid canned, bottled or frozen fruit with sweeteners, because when they are processed or juiced their nutrient and fiber content decreases and their sugar and additive content increases. |
| **VEGETABLES:** Choose raw, fresh, fresh frozen and preferably organic vegetables. Fresh raw vegetables contain no additives or preservatives and are higher in health-boosting phytochemicals. | Canned or frozen vegetables with additives can deplete essential nutrients. Also too much salt added to your vegetable intake can raise your blood pressure. Most canned foods add preservatives. |
| **GRAINS:** Are a great energy source, high in energy-releasing nutrient that feed your cells. Choose all whole grains and products containing whole grains; cereals, breads, muffins, whole-grain crackers. Whole grains are also rich in fiber which is essential for healthy digestion. | Avoid all white flour products, white rice and white pasta. |
| **DAIRY PRODUCTS:** Choose non-fat cottage cheese, unsweetened yogurt, skim milk, butter milk, rice milk, soy milk and all soy products. | Avoid soft, pasteurized or artificially colored cheeses and ice cream. These products are high in saturated fat, dyes and preservatives. |
| **NUTS:** go for all fresh, raw nuts. | Avoid salted or roasted nuts, you don't need the extra salt, fat and preservatives. |
| **GOOD FOR HEALTH** | **NOT SO GOOD FOR HEALTH** |

| **Yea!** | **Nay!** |
| --- | --- |
| **MEATS:** Choose organic skinless turkey, chicken, and lamb. Also most game meat. | Red meats are high in saturated fat. Processed-farmed meat and poultry often contain hormones and antibiotics that upset your hormonal,, immune and digestive system. |
| **EGGS:** Choose organic free-range if possible. Organic eggs won't contain the toxic hormones and antibiotics pumped into factory-produced eggs. When cooking best to boil or poach. | Avoid fried or pickled, these eggs are high in cholesterol-raising saturated fat. |
| **FISH:** Freshwater and oily fish are rich in the good fats, known as omega-3, essential for reducing cholesterol and promoting great health and well-being. | Avoid all fried fish, all shellfish, salted fish, anchovies, herring and fish canned in salt and oil. |

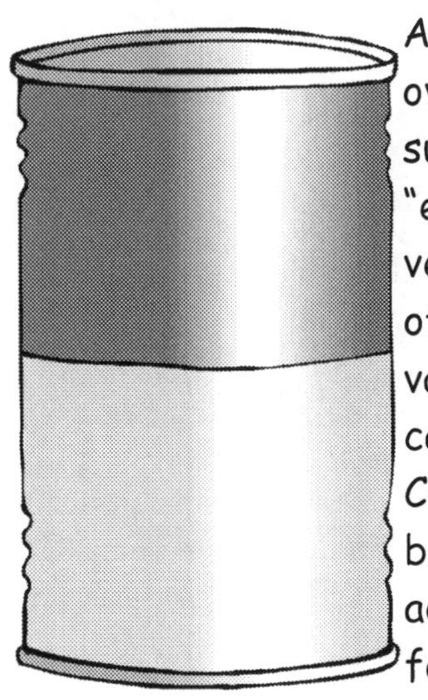

Avoid all canned foods, most are over processed, high in fats, sugar. These foods are called "empty" calories. Fruit and vegetables are fantastic source of nutrients. But their nutritional value can be depleted if they are canned or cooked in fat and salt. Canned foods are more likely to be high in toxic preservatives and additives. Most will have no life force and little nutrient content.

Its always best to purchase fresh produce, and fresh from the garden always trumps weeks of storage and transit from great distances. Even better grow your own, it would be great to have your own garden, if you have the space and time. I have for many years grown organic vegetables and fruit. And there is noting like fresh home grown foods right out of the garden. Eating fresh-picked corn or vine-ripened tomatoes is a life-altering experience.

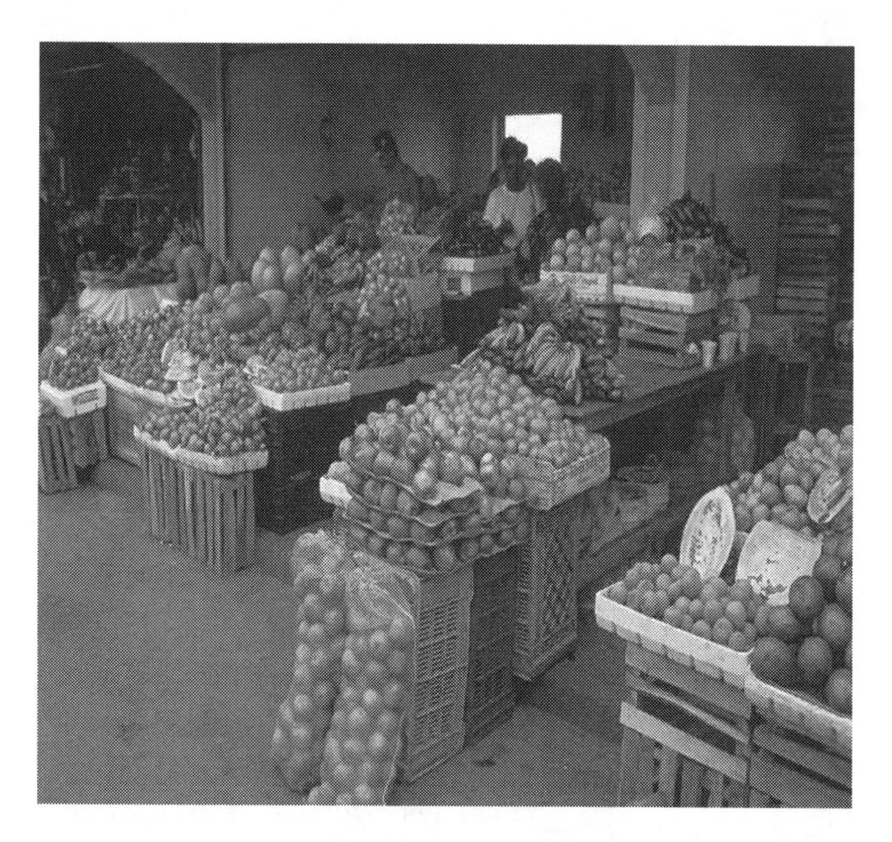

If you don't have the time needed to devote or space for growing a self-sustaining organic garden. Than try going to a farmers-market for your produce. This will give you the best chance of getting the freshes fruits and vegetables.

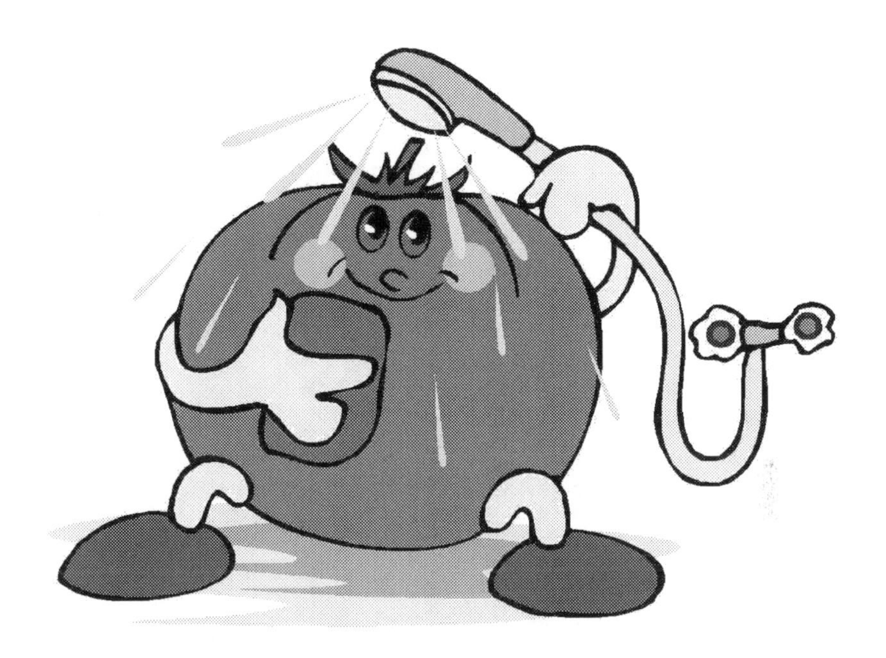

**WASHING:** Wash and scrub all fresh fruits and vegetables thoroughly under running water. Running water has an abrasive effect that soaking does not have. This will help remove any bacteria or traces of pesticide residues from the surfaces of fruits and vegetables and remove dirt from crevices. Remember not all pesticide or bacterial residues can be removed by washing,

**PEELING:** When possible peel fruits and vegetables to reduce the amount of dirt, bacteria, and pesticide residues. Discard outer leaves of leafy vegetables. Every year more people are seeing the wisdom and rewards, of eating natural foods.

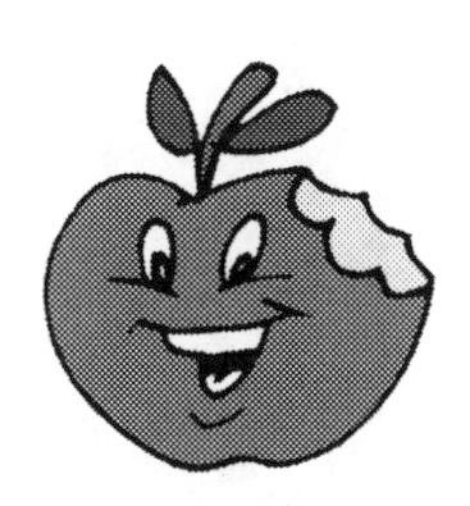

CHAPTER 3

# Choosing the right foods

# Choosing the right foods
## ( For their nutritional value )

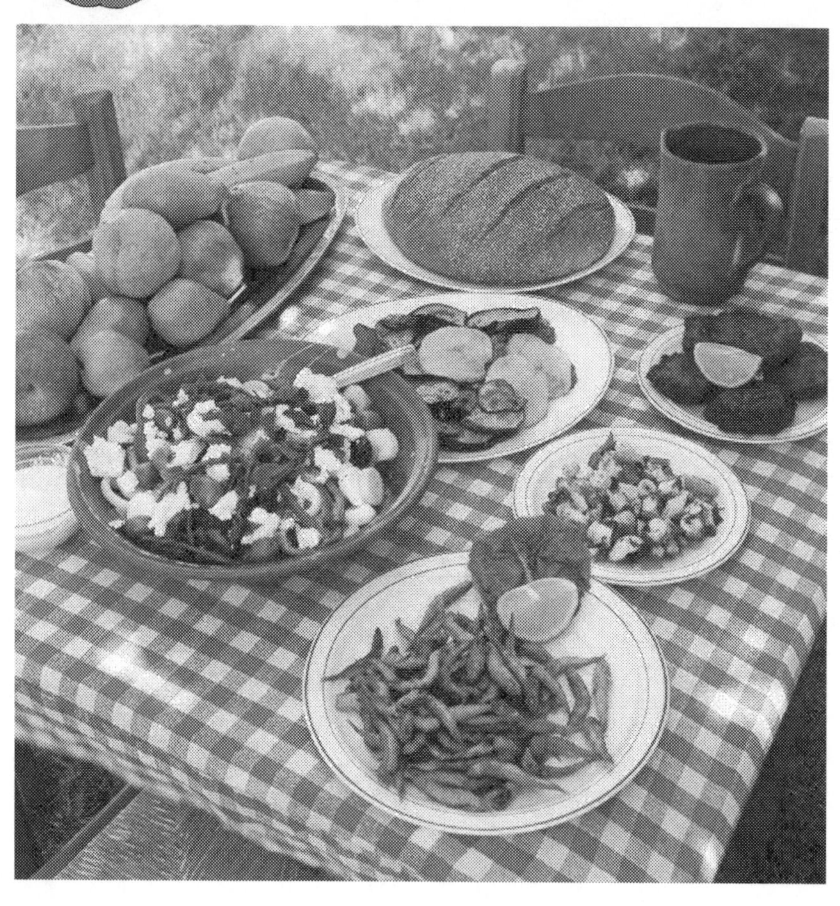

## *Good natural healthy foods*

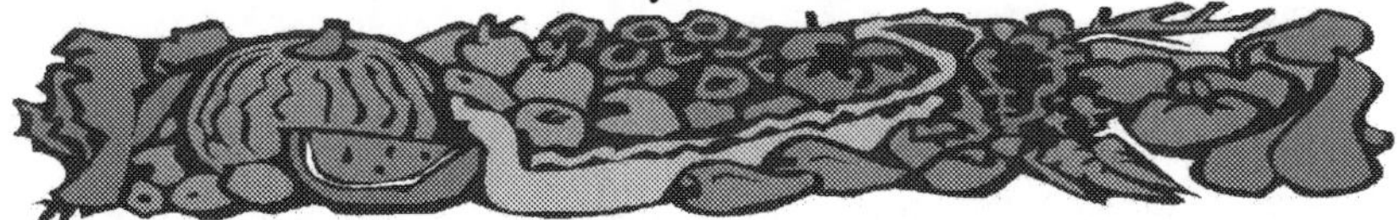

**Whole raw foods:** These foods have not been cooked, boiled, stewed, microwaved, frozen, baked or steamed. The result, they are still in their original natural state and contain all the natural enzymes. These enzymes are the life force of food which helps the digestion process. Raw vegetables, fruit, whole grains and seeds all contain food enzymes. We need an abundant supply of these enzymes to nourish our bodies, balance our metabolism and provide us with energy. Unprocessed foods are foods that have not had added chemicals or any other additives. These foods are still in their original state, the way nature grew them. There are some packaged foods that still have ingredients in their original state. But be sure to read labels.

**Organic foods:** Means foods that are free of any chemicals. These foods that are organic have been grown in soils that have not used any chemical fertilizers and/or pesticides. Remember if any kind of chemicals have been used on the produce that you eat, these chemicals, which are toxic, will enter your body cells and bloodstream. No one knows what damage they will do? There are many studies and research that show that these chemicals inside our bodies do not help our overall health.

**Carbohydrates and Protein:** Good carbohydrates are without any added refined sugar: for instance, fruits, whole grain breads, grains, rice and vegetables. There natural healthy carbs are called complex carbs. They contain naturally occurring sugars that the body can easily and slowly metabolize for balanced brain function, mood and useful energy. Vegetable protein are easy to break down in the body. Are more efficient, cheaper and healthier than protein from meat. Combining beans and grains together forms a complete protein, easy to digest and enhancing to the metabolism.

# APPLE

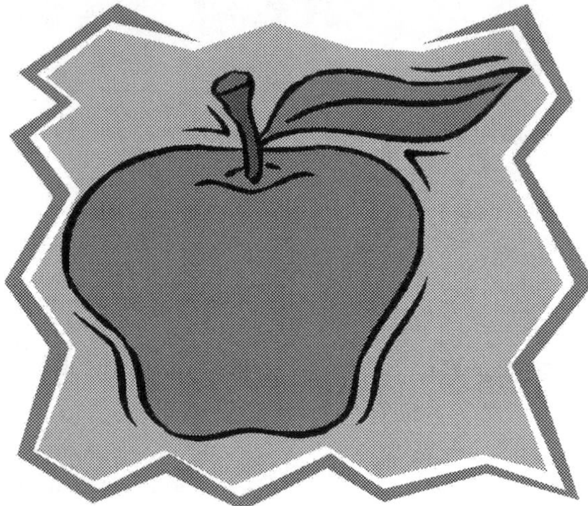

Apples
containing
fiber,
flavonoids
and vitamin C,
apples
are a healthy
addition to
your diet.

**Apple:** These tasty delights are natures candy. They Contain fiber, falconoid, and vitamin C, apples are a good healthy addition to any diet. Apples contain pectin, a fiber that flushes waste products out of the body. It also encourages beneficial bacteria to proliferate in the gut and, with quartering, helps to keep cholesterol levels down. Apples contain malic acid, to which relieves rheumatism and arthritis, and assists with energy production. Apples' vitamin C boots immunity, while their high water content dehydrates the body.

# APRICOT

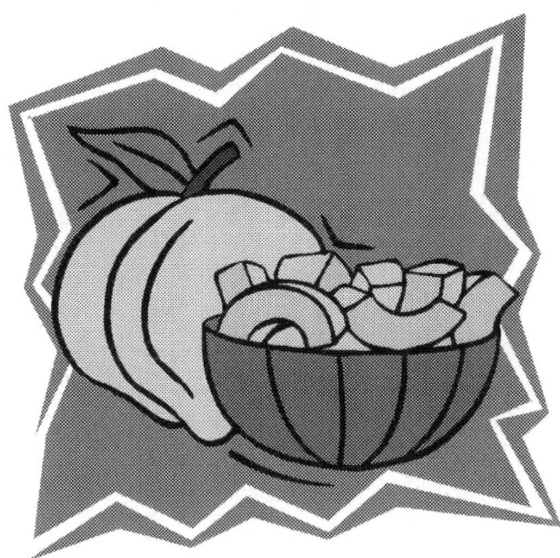

Apricot with their high carotenoid content have a wealth of nutrients.

**Apricot:** One of natures wonders, with their mouthwatering, tantalizing taste. Their high carotenoid content, apricots contain a wealth of nutrients. Beta-carotene is the most abundant antioxidant found in apricots, helping to protect the skin and lungs from oxidation damage and supporting the immune system. It prevents free radicals from damaging the eyes. In addition, apricots contain lycopene, one of the most powerful antioxidants. Lycopence is known for its ability to prevent the build-up of fatty deposits in the arteries and it has strong ant carcinogenic properties.

# AVOCADO

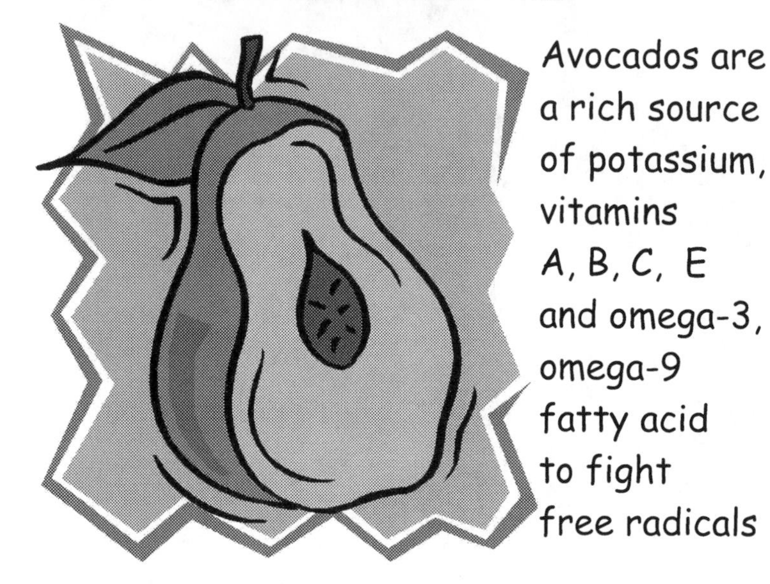

Avocados are
a rich source
of potassium,
vitamins
A, B, C, E
and omega-3,
omega-9
fatty acid
to fight
free radicals

**Avocados:** this wonderful gift from mother earth is nature at its best, they are loaded with nutrition, A, B, C, and E vitamins. Also are one of the richest sources of potassium, which is essential for healthy blood pressure and muscle contraction. They are also high in fiber.

# BANANAS

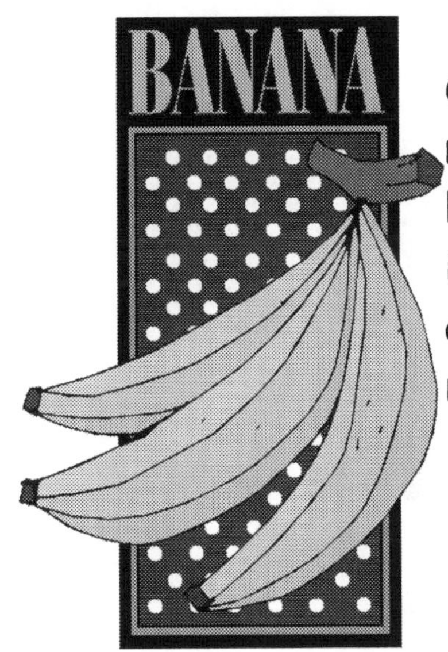


One of the
most nourishing fruits,
bananas contain many
important
anti-aging
nutrients

**Bananas:** Delightful tasty natural treat, are high in potassium, which keeps blood pressure in check and reduces the rick of heart disease. Potassium works with sodium to maintain the fluid and electrolyte balance in body cells, so bananas help to maintain healthy nerve and muscle function. They have FOS (fructo-oligo-saccharides) to help to feed good bacteria in the gut, and aid digestion. Bananas also contain tryptophan, which the body converts to serotonin to aid peaceful sleep.

# BLACKBERRIES

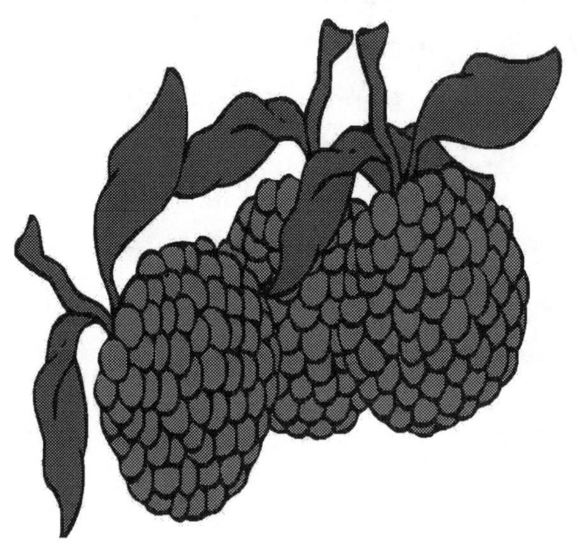

Blackberries are one of the richest low-fat sources of vitamin E

**Blackberries:** Nature's plump, sweet and juicy, blackberries are a powerhouse of nutrients, and one of the richest low-fat sources of vitamin E. Like most berries, blackberries are an excellent source of vitamin C, but what sets them apart is that they also contain good amounts of vitamin E. This helps to neutralize free radicals, which cause heart disease and premature aging of the skin. Blackberries are a natural source of salicylate, the active substance found in aspirin, which helps the body to fight infection. Some studies have shown that salicylate also has anti-carcinogenic properties.

# BLUEBERRIES

Blueberries are an excellent source of antioxidants

**Blueberries:** Blueberries these are one of my favorite fruits, they are a excellent source of antioxidants, which stave off many conditions. Blueberries are a rich source of anthocyanin, a potent antioxidant that protects against aging and improves circulation. Anthocyanin also increases the potency of vitamin C., thus supporting collagen and improving the skin. Blueberries help to improve brain function, as well as to fight eye disease. They are a good source of pectin, which lower cholesterol levels. Topically, their fruit acid content helps them to act as a gentle astringent and peeling agent.

# CANTALOUPE

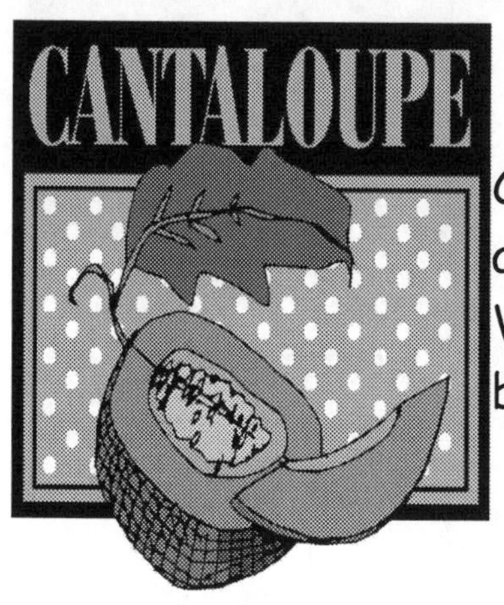


Cantaloupes
are high in antioxidants,
Vitamin C and
beta carotene

**Cantaloupe:**These succulent summer fruits are bursting with antioxidants to fight off free radicals. Cantaloupe are very rich in vitamin C and beta carotene, both of which are naturally aid cell repair and growth, as well as supporting the immune and circulatory systems. Cantaloupes also contain potassium, which can lower high blood pressure and bad LDL cholesterol. With their high water content, cantaloupes help to detoxify the body.

# CHERRIES

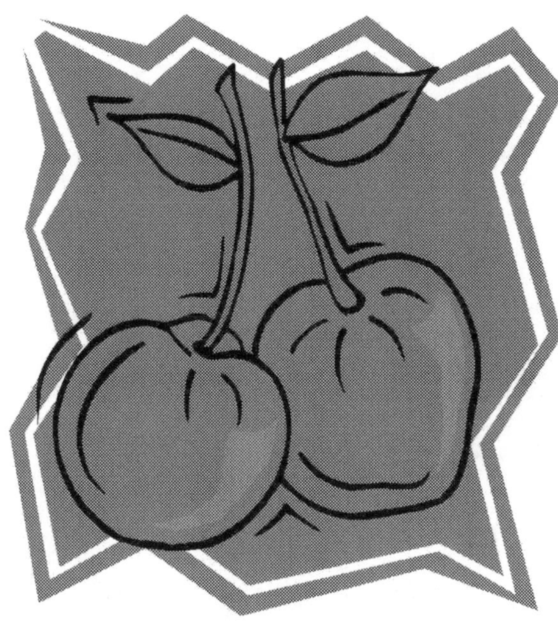

Cherries are
high in
falconoid
as
anthocyanins,
which the body
uses to help
immunity

**Cherries:** Cherries are packed with antioxidants. Cherries are high in falconoid as anthocyanins, which the body uses to help boot immunity. They contain quartering, a strong anti-inflammatory substance, which helps to relieve painful joints and protects against eye disease. Cherries are rich in the phytochemical ellagic acid, which has anti-carcinogenic properties and vitamin C, which strengthens collagen and in addition, vitamin Cacids to fight viruses and bacteria.

# LEMONS

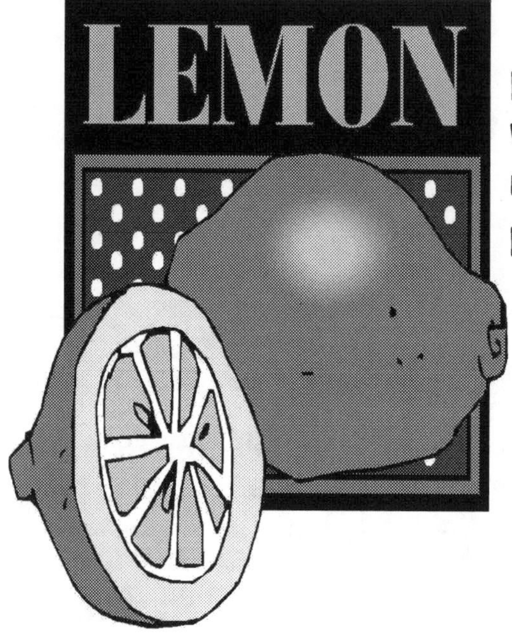


provide a wealth of nutritional properties

**Lemons:** Years ago lemons were used by seaman to fight off scurvy while out at sea. Lemons have a very high level of vitamin C. Which means that they are vital for healthy body. Lemons are also great source of bioflavonoids, such as quercetin, which boost the effects of vitamin C, lemons are particularly important for healthy blood vessels and prevent varicose veins. Lemon juice inhibits bacterial growth and is astringent, strengthening, and toning.

# ORANGES

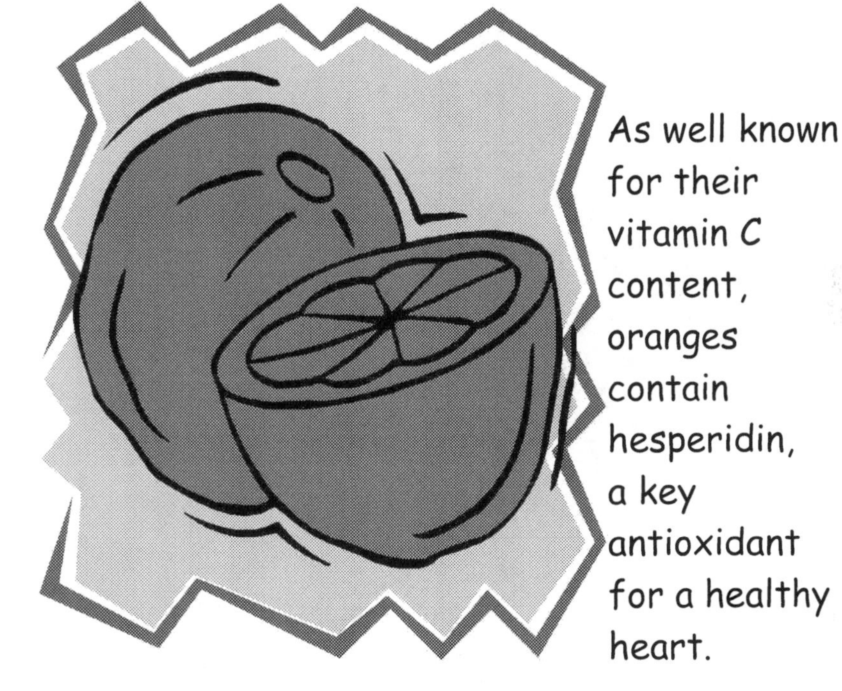

As well known for their vitamin C content, oranges contain hesperidin, a key antioxidant for a healthy heart.

**Orange:** Other one of nature's wonders, They are very rich in in vitamin C, oranges help to maintain healthy, skin, helps prevent eye problems, and stop free radicals from clogging up your arteries. Which is a a factor for heart disease. They also protect the heart further by raising healthy HDL cholesterol and lowing bad LDL cholesterol. They provide natural sugars to boost flagging energy levels, high in fiber and are even reputed to reduce cellulite.

# STRAWBERRIES

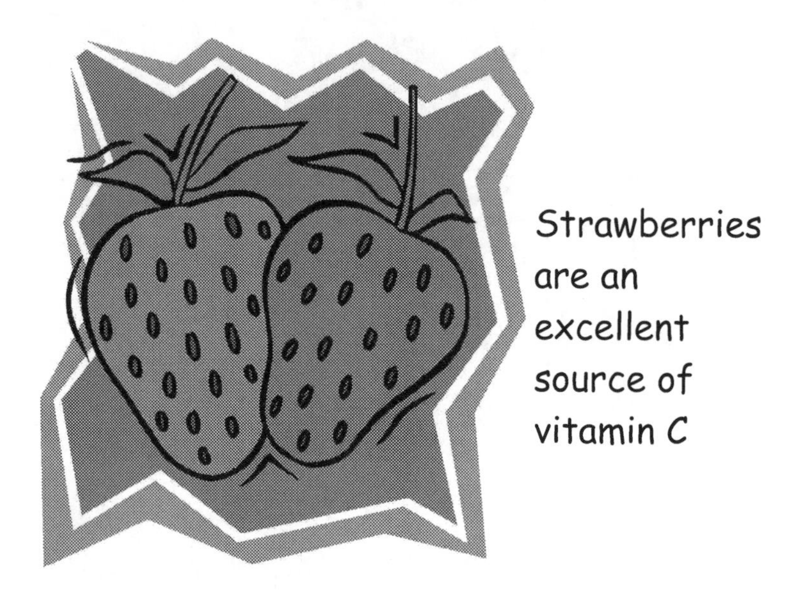


**Strawberries:** Who doesn't love Strawberries, they are so succulent, and an excellent source of vitamin C, which is essential for the manufacture of collagen, a protein that helps to maintain the structure of the skin. Vitamin also plays an important role in healing wounds and can ward off gingivitis, a gum disease that can affect some adults. Strawberries contain ellagic acid, a phytochemical that has powerful anti-carcinogenic properties.

# GRAPES

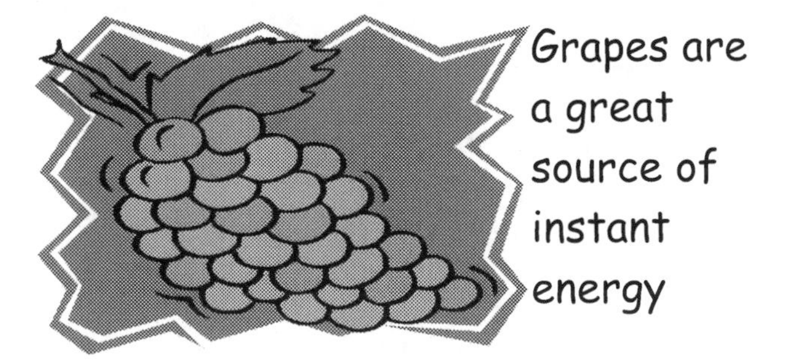


**Grapes:** A great succulent source of instant energy. Grapes contain an enormous number of compounds that are uniquely nourishing, thus giving them a reputation as a food for convalescents. This aromatic fruit can prevent and help to treat any number of conditions, from anemia and fatigue to arthritis, varicose veins and rheumatism. Full of powerful antioxidant including astringent tannins, flavones, and anthocyanins, grapes help to prevent bad LDL cholesterol from oxidizing and blood from clotting, and therefore protect the heart and circulatory system. High in both water and fiber, grapes are a great aid for detoxifying the gut and liver. Black grapes also contain quartering which helps to minimize inflammation, aiding the cardiovascular system further, as well as promoting healthy digestion. Grape has been dried to make raisins. Dynamos of concentrated nutrients, raisins are full of fiber and exceptionally high energy, are rich in the minerals iron, potassium, selenium

# RASPBERRIES

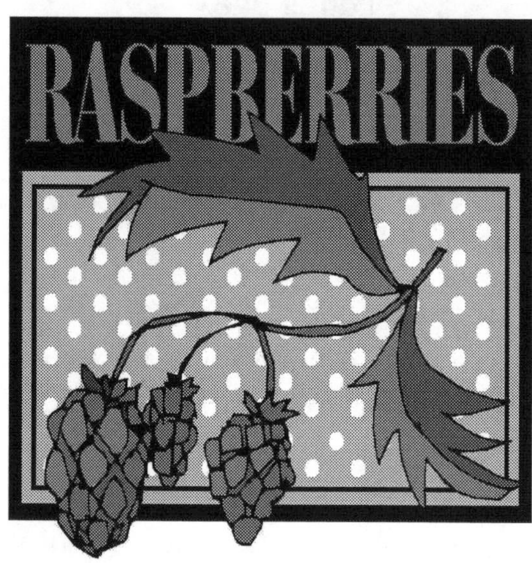


Raspberries have a very high C content

**Raspberries:** Other succulent fruit from mother earth, Raspberries have a high vitamin C content that boosts immunity and can help to prevent everything from heart disease to eye problems. Raspberries also contain ellagic acid, which is anti-carcinogenic and prevents adverse cellular changes. The anthocyanins in raspberries have anti-inflammatory properties, thus protecting from conditions such as arthritis. They are one of the top fruit sources of fiber, therefore improving digestion

# PINEAPPLE

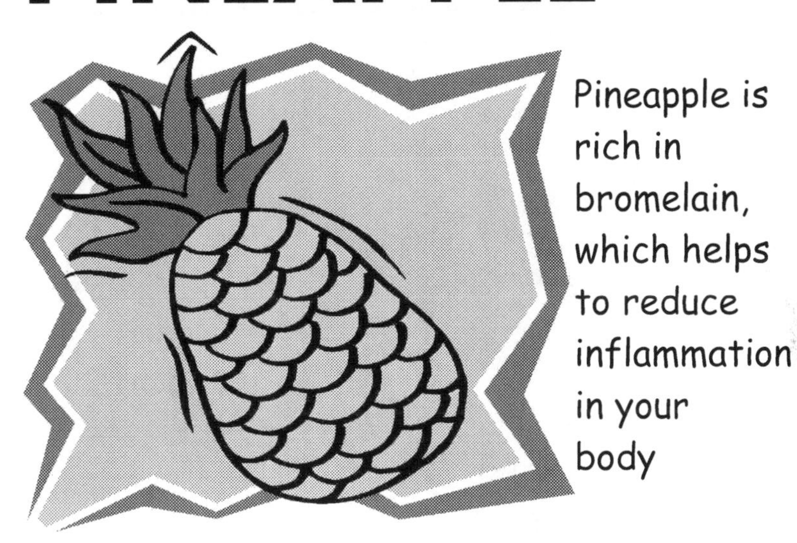

Pineapple is rich in bromelain, which helps to reduce inflammation in your body

**Pineapple:** What a wonderful delight from the earth's bounty, the main benefits in pineapple come from bromelain, which is an effective anti-inflammatory, making exceptionally good for joint problems. Also pineapple are high in vitamin C, they also support the immune system and defend against free radicals, which can cause premature aging. They are an excellent source of a number of enzymes important for antioxidant defenses and energy production.

# POMEGRANATE

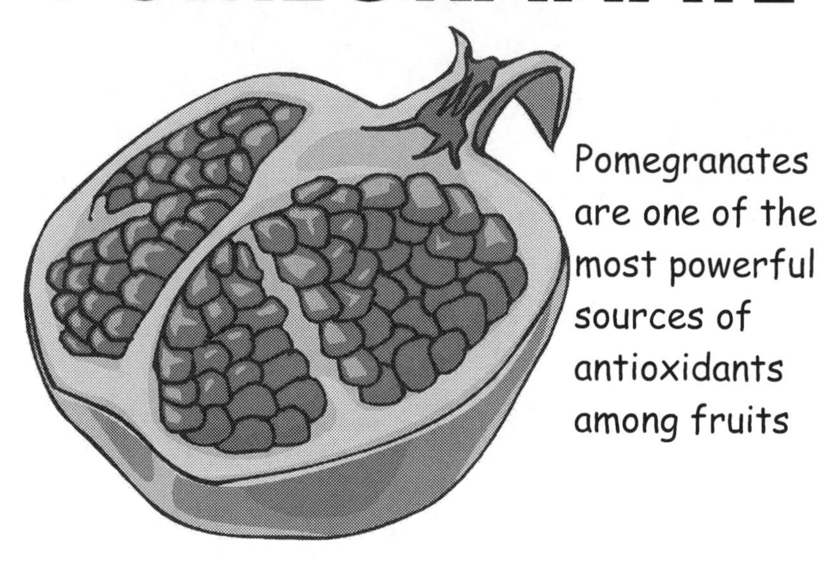

Pomegranates are one of the most powerful sources of antioxidants among fruits

**Pomegranates:** Can't say enough about this amazing food from nature, they are extremely rich in ellagic acid, pomegranates have anti-carcinogenic and anti-heart disease properties. Antioxidants in pomegranates protect against free-radical damage, including to the skin, and also keeps the arteries clear. Antioxidant chemicals also protect the skin from sun damage.

# RHUBARB

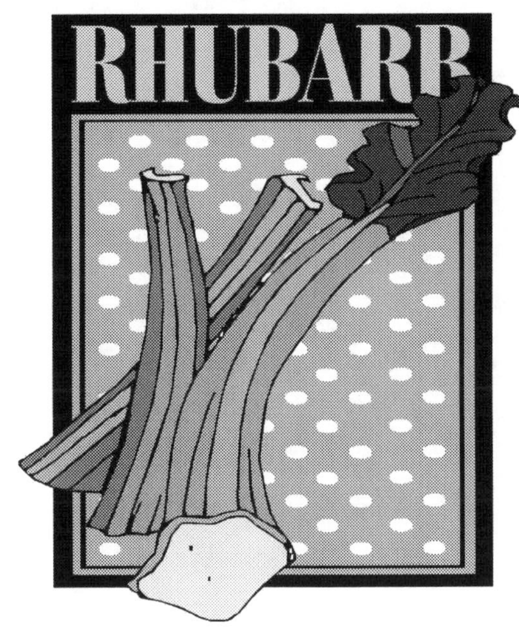


Rhubarb is
a great source
of dietary
fiber as
well as
vitamin C
and minerals

**Rhubarb:** Have you ever had a rhubarb pie, one of the delights of life. Rhubarb is full of fiber, and acts as a natural food laxative, keeping the digestive system in great condition and helps to lower cholesterol and thus preventing heart disease. It is also high in calcium for bones, potassium to keep blood pressure down and protect the heart

# PUMPKIN

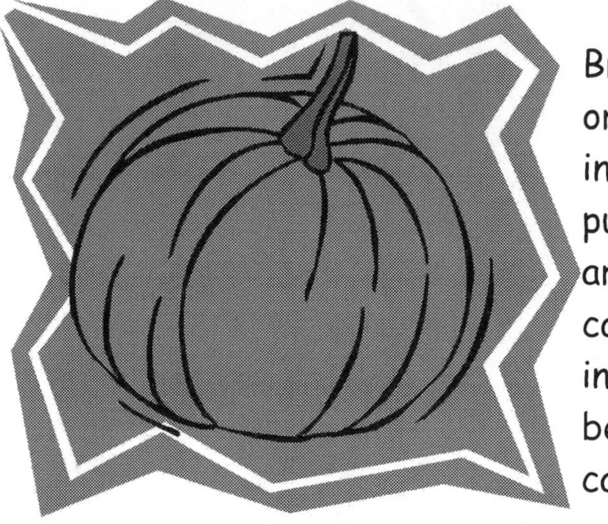

Bright orange in color, pumpkins are rich in carotenoids including beta-carotene

**Pumpkins:** What can one say about this fall delight. Not only are they good for you, but fun for the kids, lets not forget the jack-o-lantern. Pumpkin has high levels of arytenoids and antioxidants, including beta-carotene, which can help prevent heart disease and eye problems. Pumpkins contain plenty of vitamin C which boosts immunity.

# ASPARAGUS

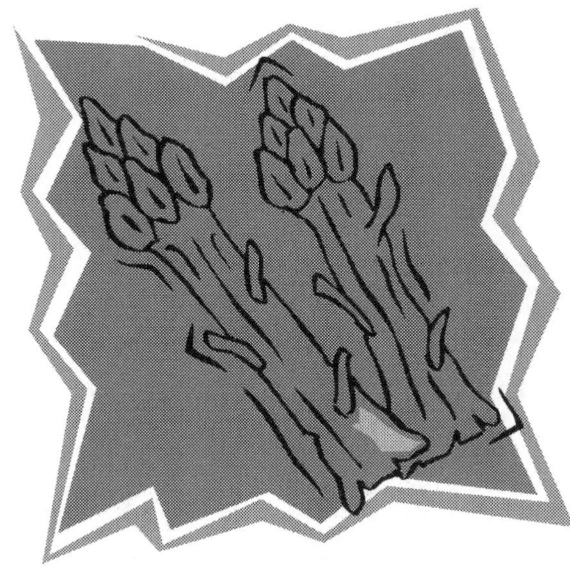

Asparagus contains vitamin E to keep the skin and heart healthy

**Asparagus:** Asparagus is a fantastic vegetable of the earth, and a great source of foliate, which is said to prevent damage to the arteries that supply blood to the heart and brain. Foliate has demonstrated anti-carcinogenic properties. Asparagus contain asparagines, which along with its high potassium and low sodium content makes it an excellent diuretic and clearer. The vegetable is also high in vitamin E to protect the heart and keep the brain young

# BEETS

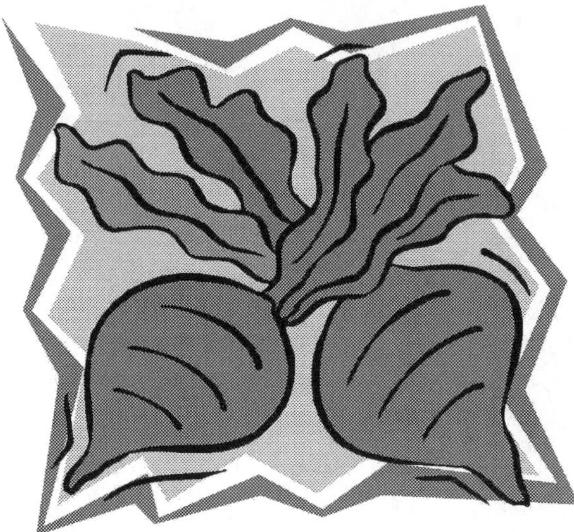

Beets are loaded with nutrients that boost the body's natural defenses

**Beets:** I like some sliced beets on my summer salad. Beets are loaded with nutrients, containing the powerful antioxidant, which gives beets their deep red hue. These vegetables purify the blood and have anti-carcinogenic properties. Beets boost the body's natural defenses in the liver, regenerating immune cells and helping to lower cholesterol levels. Beets contain silica, which is vital for healthy skin, hair, fingernails, ligaments, tendons and bones.

# PEPPERS

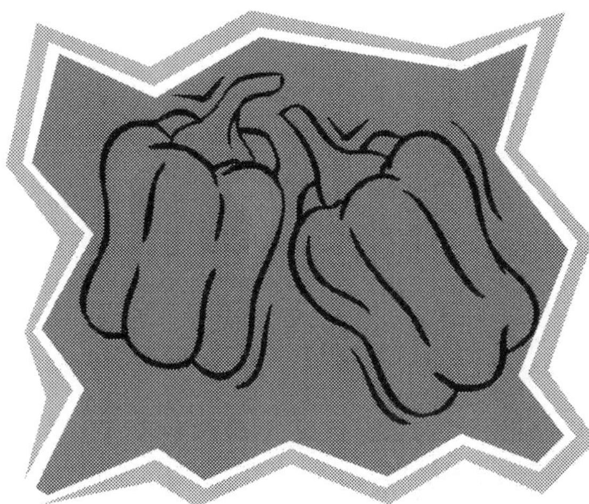

Bell peppers are a a rich source of vitamin C, and antibiotics

**Bell Peppers:** Are so great in so many ways, raw, cooked, grilled, etc. Peppers are packed with vitamin C, which helps to fight almost every aspect of aging process, including deterioration of the skin structure and damage to the arteries. Vitamin C is said to quash carcinogenic free radicals, and to protect against memory problems and eye disease. It is a potent immunity booster. Red bell pepper is rich source of lycopene, another renowned anti-carcinogenic nutrient.

# BROCCOLI

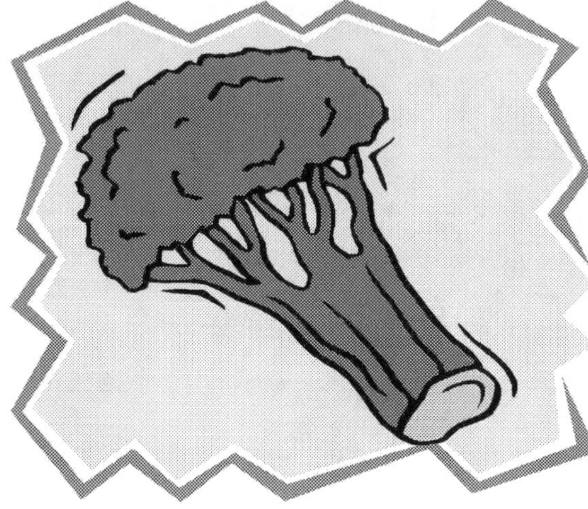

Broccoli is
rich in
beta-carotene
and a great
source
of vitamin C

**Broccoli:** Broccoli with its high levels of arytenoids,especially beta-carotene, has powerful anti-carcinogenic properties and has been associated with lower rates of both heart and eye disease. As broccoli can increase vitamin A in the body, it also helps to improve various skin conditions. It is a great source of vitamin C, which helps to boost immunity. Broccoli contains calcium, which starves off osteoporosis and fiber, which keeps the digestive system working smoothly. one of the characteristic of this plant is it contains enzyme inhibitors that interfere with the digestion and utilization of nutrients in the diet. They must be cooked or steamed to destroy the anti - nutritional factors.

# CABBAGE

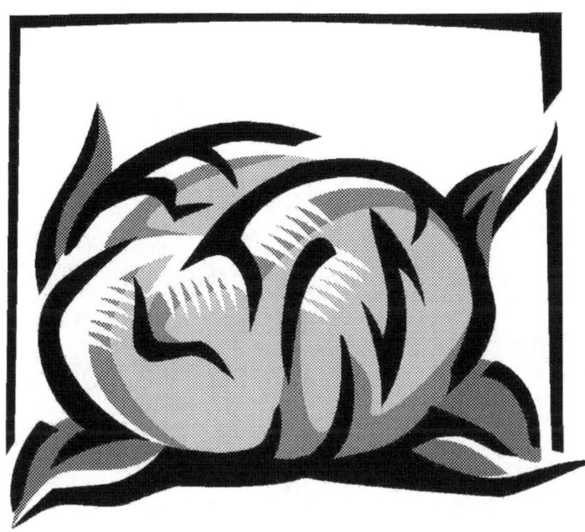

Cabbage contains a range of sulphuous substances and other nutrients to keep us healthy

**Cabbage:** This vegetable gets looked over by a lot of people, but cabbage is rich in sulphur, which protects the liver and has anti-carcinogenic properties; Sulphur is a constituent of keratin. Also has collagen, vitamin C in cabbage mops up free radicals. It also contains vitamin B3, folate, calcium and potassium.

# CARROTS

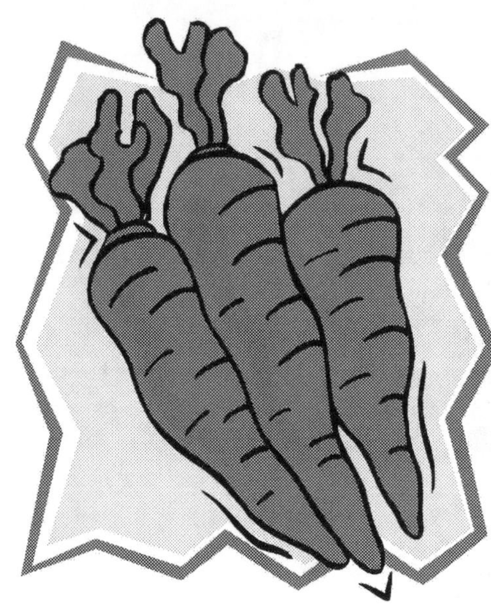

Carrots are rich in Beta-carotene, which the body converts into vitamin A

**Carrots:** This is a great vegetable, carrots with their beta-carotene, which the body converts into vitamin A, is especially important for eye health. It's a great benefit to the skin, and the immune and digestive system. Along with alpha-carotene, it is anti-carcinogenic and helps to reduce the risk of heart disease. Carrots are loaded with fiber and water, which cleanse the liver, boost detoxification, and plump out the skin to stave off wrinkles. The vitamin C and silica content of carrots is also valuable for keeping the skin youthful.

# CELERY

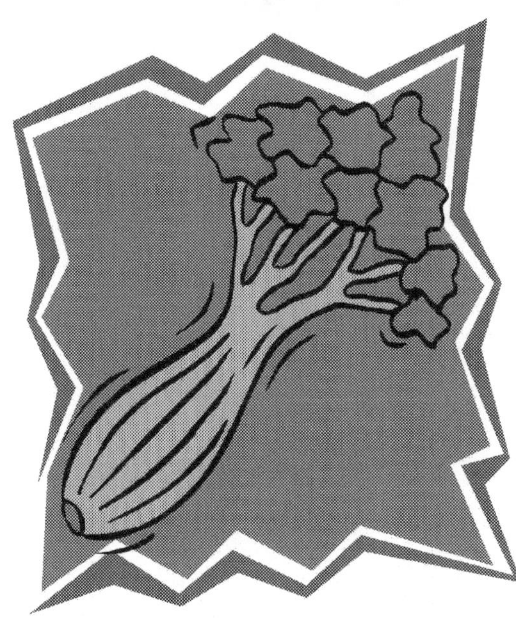

Celery contains very few calories, this aids weight loss and keeps us looking great

**Celery:** Did you know that you can burn as many calories crewing celery as you get from the plant, that is why it is a good vegetable to eat when on a weight loss program. Not only that, but celery has a high water content acting as a diuretic, helping to eliminate puffy hands, ankles and feet. Celery is also excellent for the body's detoxifying processes, including cleaning of the liver.

# CUCUMBERS

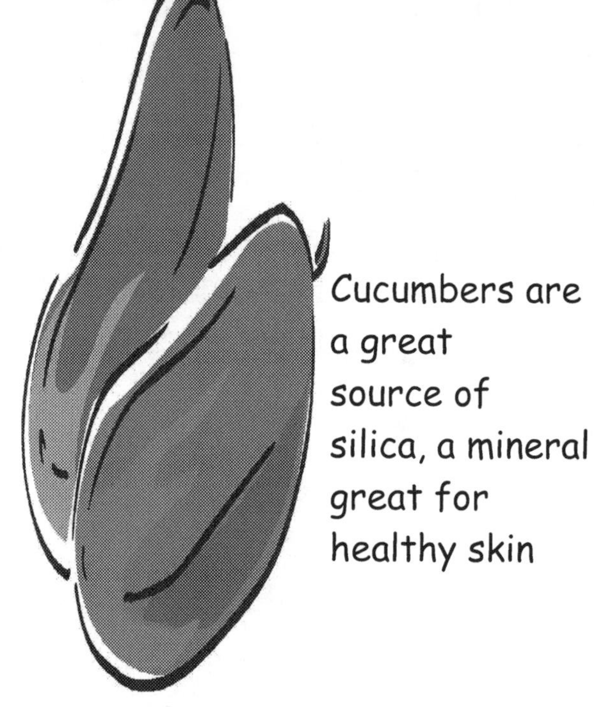

Cucumbers are a great source of silica, a mineral great for healthy skin

**Cucumbers:** Cucumber are great with your salad Cucumber helps to maintain a youthful appearance, thanks to its hydrating and anti-inflammatory properties. Ingested, the high water and balanced mineral content make it one of the best diuretics. Also a very rich source of silica, a mineral needed for healthy skin, bone and connective tissue. Silica also helps in preventing cardiovascular disease and osteoporosis.

# KALE

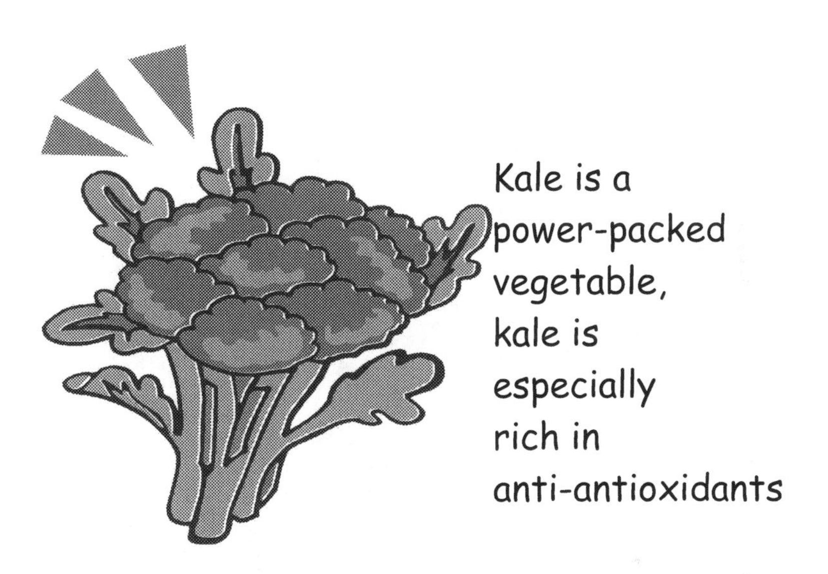


**Kale:** Other natural wonder, Kale is high in B-vitamins and arytenoids and a host of minerals. Its vitamin B6 and B12 content helps to boost brain power and prevent memory loss. Loaded with beta-carotene, it is also a very good source of lutein, a carotenoid that helps to prevent eye disease. Kale is a great source of calcium for bones and silica for the skin, hair, teeth and nails. Silica counteracts the negative effects of aluminum in the body.

# MUSHROOM

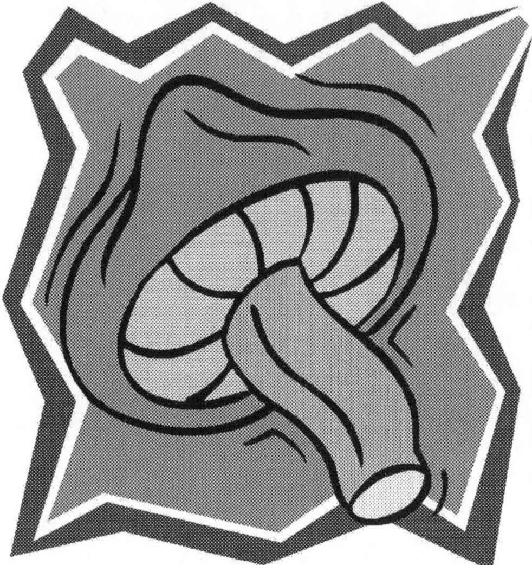

Mushrooms are rich in vitamin E and selenium. They also have more protein than most vegetables

**Mushrooms:** Most people do not think about mushrooms as a healthy food, but they are a rich source of vitamin E, selenium and potassium which helps to maintain and protect against heart disease. Mushroom also boost the immunity system.

# ONIONS

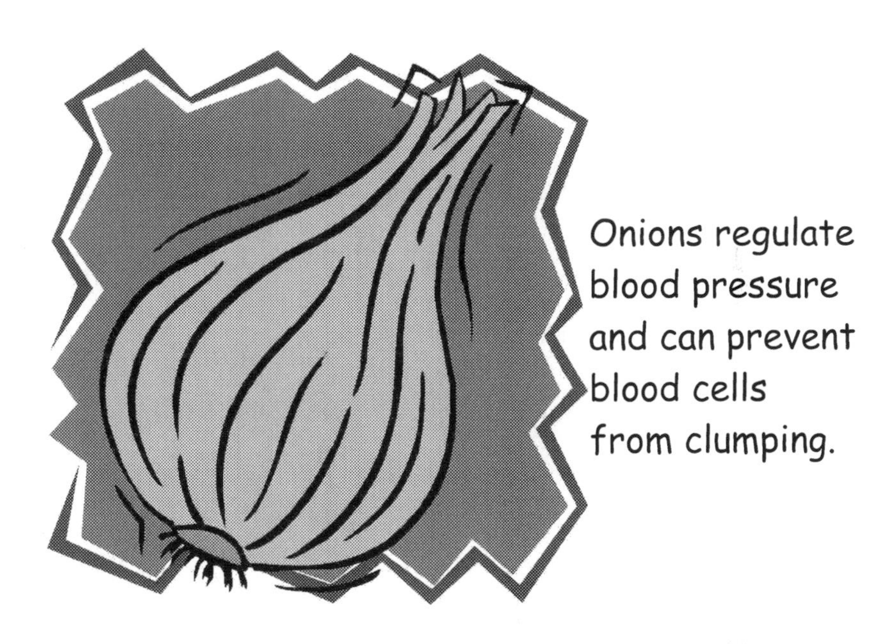


**Onions:** A very versatile food, raw, grill, stewed, etc. It is a cousin of garlic, and contains powerful antioxidant. Onions regulate blood pressure and can prevent blood cells from clumping. Also there is a great source of quartering, selenium, sulphur, which acts as an anti-inflammatory, boosts immunity, and cleanses the liver, starves off sun damage.

# SWEET POTATO

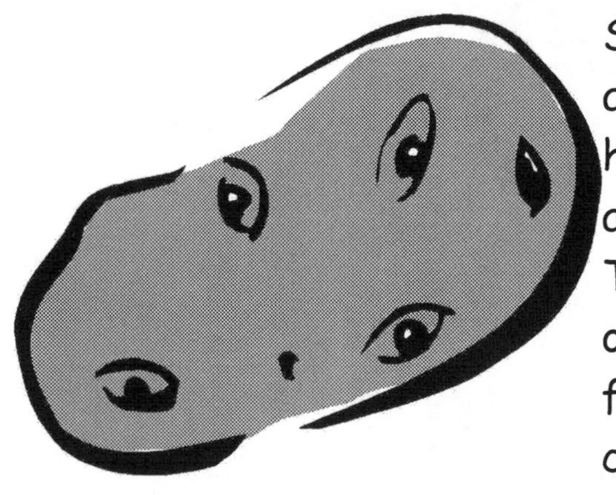

Sweet potatoes are extremely high in antioxidant. They are one of the few foods that contain both C and E vitamins.

**Sweet potato:** This is other food people don't think of as a healthy source of nutritional value, They look at it as something they eat on the holidays, Thanksgiving and Christmas. But they are extremely high in antioxidants. Orange sweet potatoes are rich in beta-carotene, which keeps the eyes, skin and lungs in good health, and supports the immune system. They also contain vitamin B6, which preserves memory and protects the heart.

# RADISHES

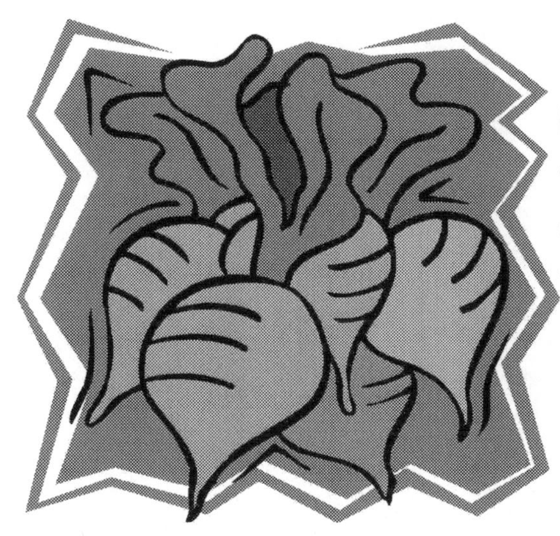

Radishes are a valuable source of potassium to keep the heart healthy

**Radishes:** A great food for salad. Radishes are rich in sulphur, which is essential for healthy skin, hair and nails, and has anti-carcinogenic properties. Assisting the body in ridding itself of toxins, which help to treat gall bladder and liver problems. Radishes are a valuable source of potassium to keep the heart healthy, calcium to prevent osteoporosis, vitamin C to fight against eye problems, and selenium to boost immunity.

# SPINACH

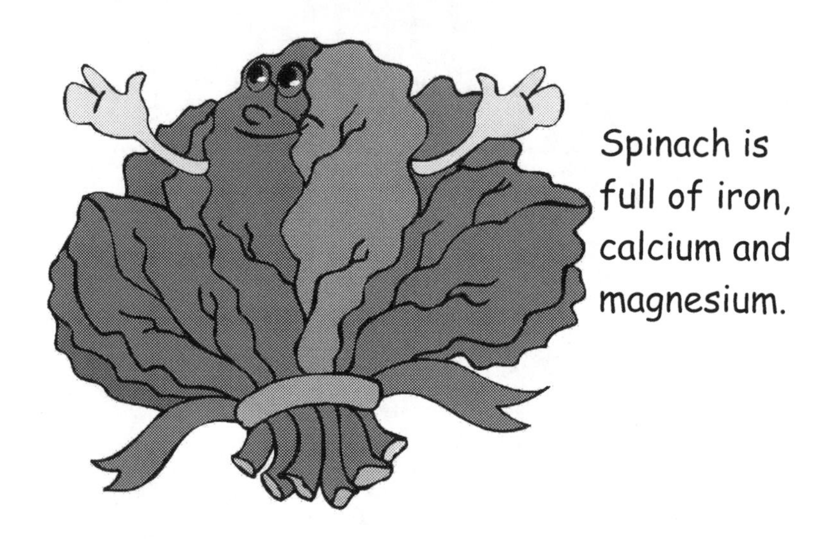


**Spinach:** What a great food, Pop-eye knew! Spinach is full of iron, calcium and magnesium. Is excellent for oxygenating the blood, generating energy, and preventing anemia. Starves off osteoporosis, and also relaxes and dilates blood vessels and keeps the muscles flexible.

# TOMATOES

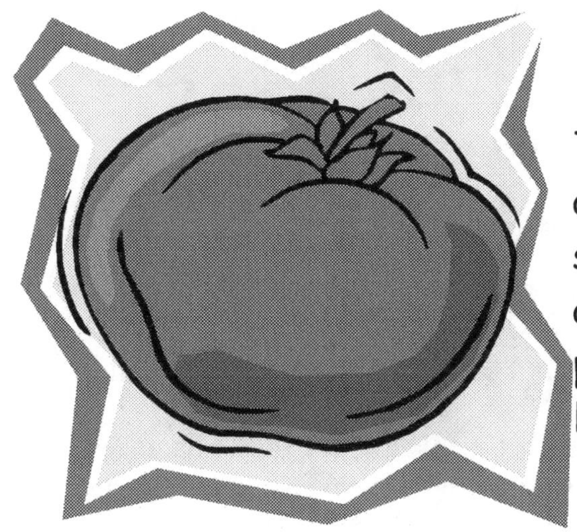

Tomatoes are a great source of arytenoids, particularly lycopene

**Tomatoes:** The tomato everyone's favorite summer fruit. Eating them raw, on a sandwich, in a salad, etc. Tomatoes are a great source of arytenoids, particularly lycopene, which neutralizes free radicals before they can cause damage, therefore, staving off heart attacks. Studies indicate that lycopene has twice the anti-carcinogenic punch of beta-carotene. In addition, tomatoes contain some iron and are high in vitamin C.

# NUTS

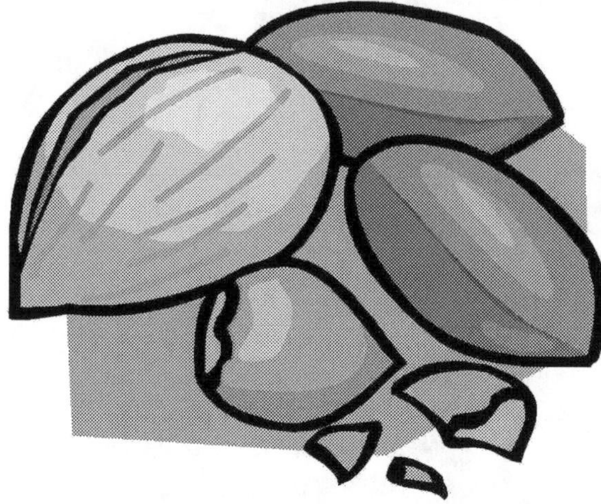

Nuts are a great snack food, providing many nutrients as well a healthy oil.

***"In a nut-shell"*** These little delights are full of healthy nutrient such as vitamin B6, E, potassium, magnesium, copper, zinc, omega-3 and omega-6 fatty acids.

**Almonds** contains a host of oils and nutrients such as fiber, almonds have more fiber than any other nut, also a great source of calcium, protein.

**Brazil nut** are rich in "good" fats and are full of selenium, and a good source of omega -3 and omega-6 essential fatty acids, which keeps us healthy.

**Cashew nut** seeds of the Brazilian *Cashew* apple These nuts are full of healthy fats and protein.

**Walnuts** are a great healthy food, providing many nutrients.

**Peanuts** are full of heart-healthy nutrients and provide more protein than any other nut.

# SEEDS

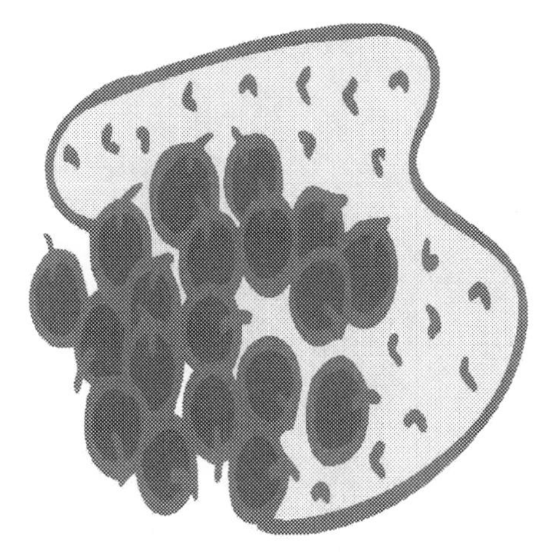

Although small, seeds are powerhouses in nutrition

Although small, *seeds* are powerhouses in nutritional essential nutrients for an alert mind, a healthy heart, and an efficient immune system and central to good-looking skin.

**Pumpkin seeds** are tasty and nutritious, pumpkin seeds are full of essential fatty acids and micronutrients.

**Flax seeds** has a nutty, sweet taste, flax seeds are loaded with essential fats for a youthful body and brain.

**Sunflower seeds** are full of vitamin E, omega-6 essential fatty acids and monousaturated fats, which helps the skin elastic and minimize heart disease.

# GRAINS

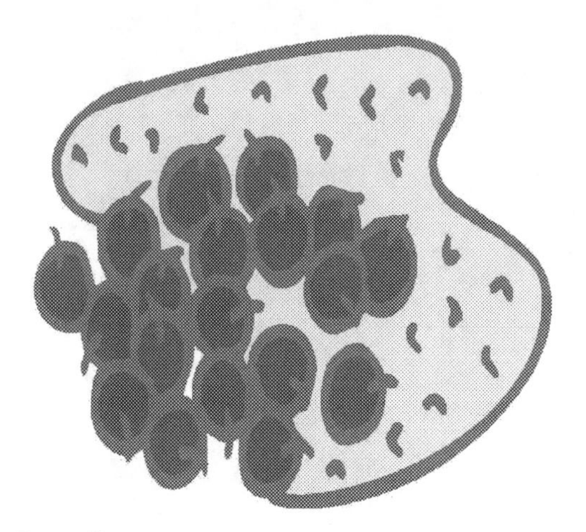

*Grains are great for the heart, grains are also full of antioxidants to fight damaging free radicals and the effects of aging*

**Barley** is the oldest cultivated cereal, and was used widely as a strengthening food. Barley is one of the best sources of the antioxidant tocotrienol, which research have show to be even more potent than some forms of vitamin E.

**Brown rice** is an excellent source of fiber, which keeps the digestive system in good health and helps to lower cholesterol in the blood.

**Oats** are very versatile and are useful for preventing heart disease and boosting immunity. As well as being a great source of energy-giving carbohydrates, oats are high in fiber, there maintaining steady blood sugar levels and preventing diabetes and lowering cholesterol.

**Whole wheat** a staple food in the western diet, wheat is protein-rich, providing B-vitamins and minerals.

# BEANS

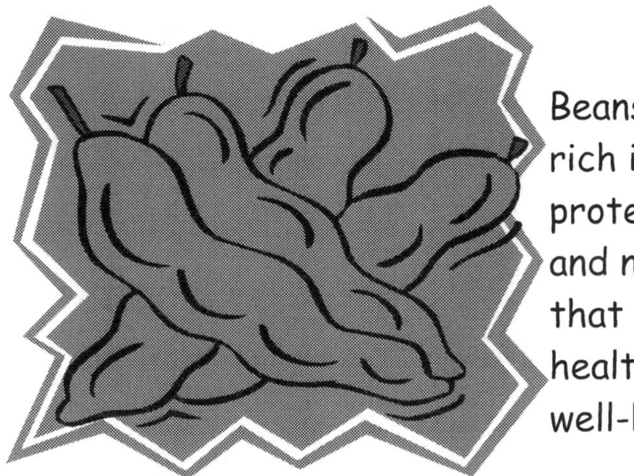

Beans are rich in protein, fiber, and nutrients that maintain health and well-being

**Garbanzo** Also known as chickpeas, are a great source of protein, which is vital for the healthy repair of our cells, their rich vitamin E content boosts the immune system.

**Kidney and Navy beans** these beans are high in fiber, which is vital for keeping cholesterol levels down and aiding digestion. Also an excellent source of protein.

**Soybeans** eating a diet rich in this versatile legume is believed to help to prevent heart disease, as well at to promote good health and longevity. The soybean is central to the diet of the Japanese, who have the longest life spans in the world.

# EGGS

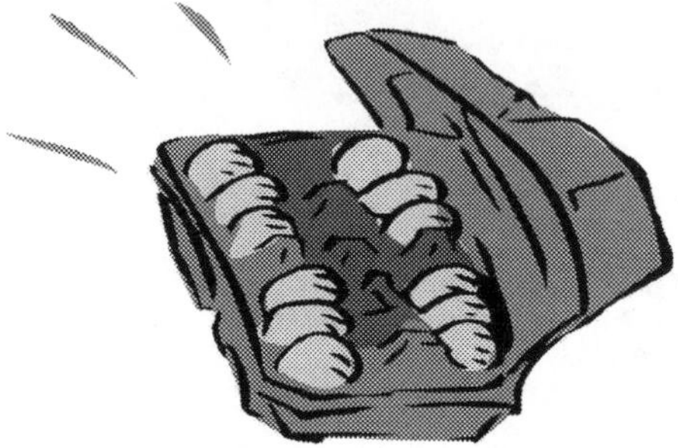

The egg
is a fantastic,
food busting
with nutrient

**Eggs:** Many of us worry about the apparently high cholesterol content of eggs, but studies suggest this might be unfounded as the cholesterol in eggs does not circulate in the blood. In fact, of the 5 grams of fat contained in an egg, most is mono unsaturated, which is the type that helps to lower the risk of heart disease. Both the whites and yolks, pack a powerful punch when it comes to nutrients. Very high in protein, eggs have all eight essential amino acids, thus helping to make up the building blocks for the entire body. Benefiting everything from bones to muscles, and hair to skin. Eggs are also a very high source of zinc and vitamins A,  B, D, and E. Vitamin A supports vision, Vitamin D promotes strong bones, and vitamin E benefit's the heart, zinc will boost immunity and is vital for the production of collagen. They also have high lecithin content, an important brain food, contributing to memory and concentration. Also helps to keep a healthy emotional state. Egg yolk is the richest known source of chiline, which makes up cell membranes, helping the body convert fats to acetylcholine, an important memory molecule in the brain.

# CHICKEN

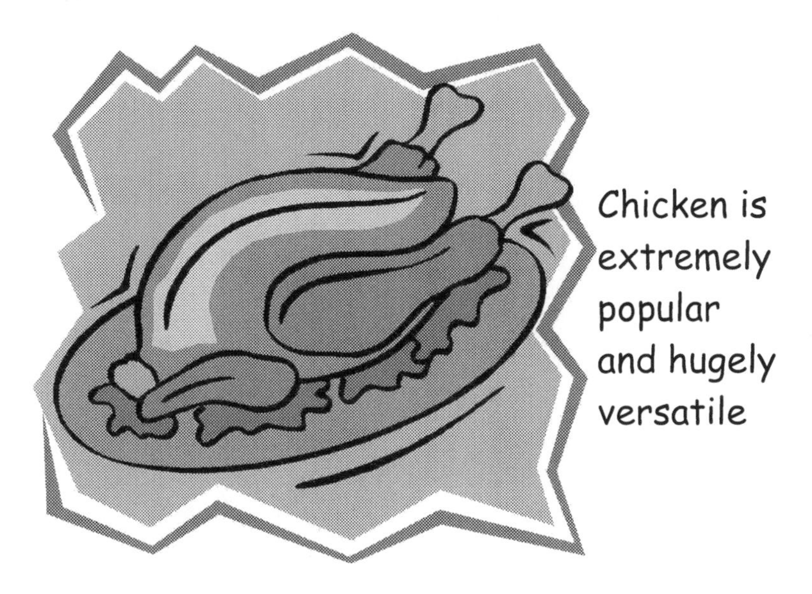

Chicken is extremely popular and hugely versatile

**Chicken:** Chicken is extremely popular and hugely versatile, bursting with health giving nutrients. Is a great source of protein, contributing to the growth and repair of body cells, and with the skin removed, is low in fat. It's high in selenium, also contains iron and zinc to boost energy levels and immunity. There is twice as much in dark meat as in the breast. The breast is particularly high in vitamin B6, which protects the heart.

# FISH

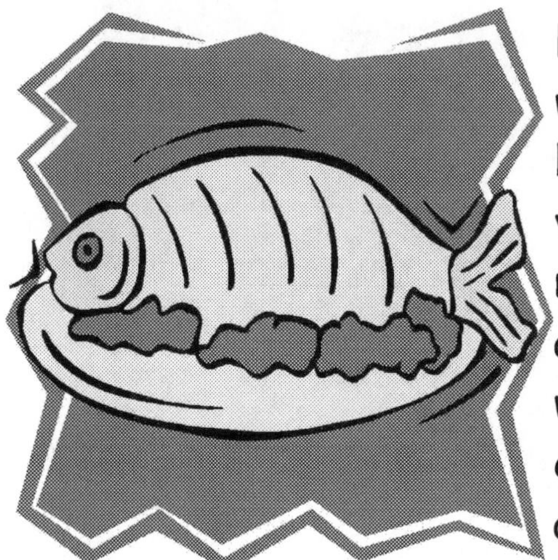

Fish are packed with health-boosting vitamins and minerals and fatty acids, which are with life enhancing attributes

**Herring** is rich in omega-3 and many vitamins, the fat-soluble vitamins A, D, and e as well as the water-soluble B vitamins, thus preventing arthritic conditions and reducing the risk of heart disease.

**Haddock** contains several B-vitamins to boost brain power and fight fatigue. It's especially rich in folate, which helps to protect against heart disease.

**Salmon** is one of nature's greatest sources of omega-3 fatty acids as well as DHA (docosahexaenoic), both are renowned for reducing heart disease. These essential fatty acids have powerful anti-inflammatory properties, making them useful for arthritic conditions. DHA is important for the brain and nervous system.

# HONEY

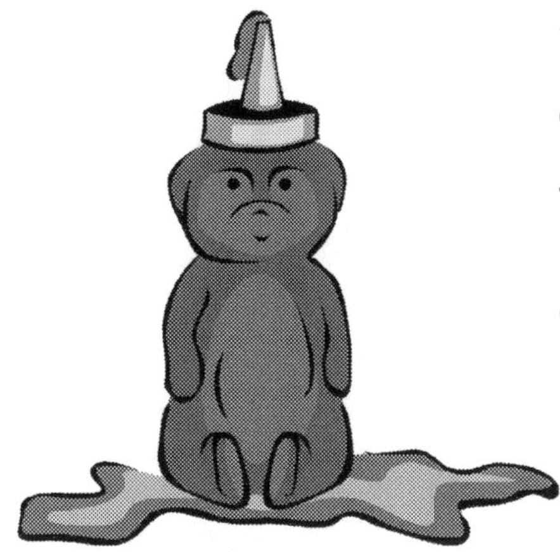

The bee by-products, essentially those substances produced by bees, have exceptional healing powers. They include royal jelly, bee pollen

**Honey:** Mother earth's natural sweetener. Honey is best known as an energy food, widely used as a natural sweetener, honey is composed of 79 percent sugar. The rest comprises water and small amounts of B vitamins, calcium, copper, iron, magnesium, phosphorus, potassium, sodium and zinc. Used topically, honey is a humectant, attracting and retaining water, which keeps the skin soft and supple.

# WATER

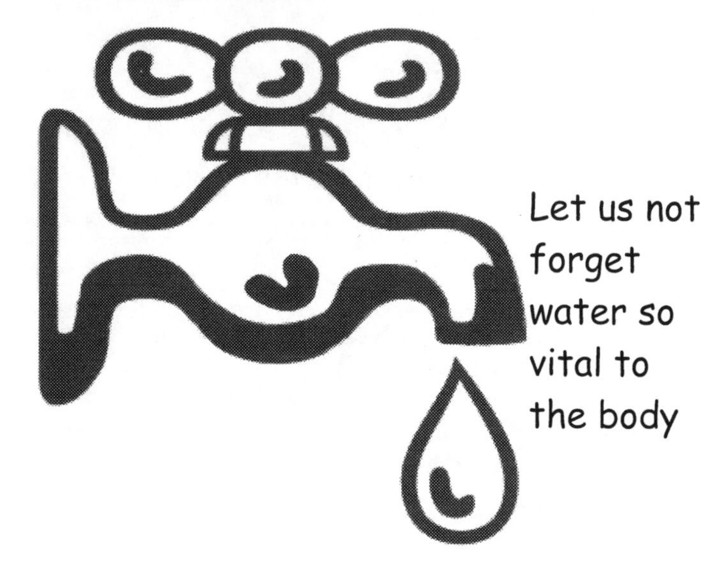


**Water** Let us not forget water so vital to the body. This is not surprising, given the average adult is made up of about 70% water. Water is vital for the blood circulation and for chemical reactions in the digestive and metabolic processes. It carries nutrients and oxygen to cells through the blood, thus stimulating the organs. We need water to breathe our lungs must be moist to take in oxygen. Water also regulates and controls the natural pH balance. Revitalizing, hydrating, oxygenating, and detoxifying. Water is vital to all plant life. Watering your plants during the growing season is essential for healthy plants. Especially in hot weather and when plants are ripening.

# REMEMBER!

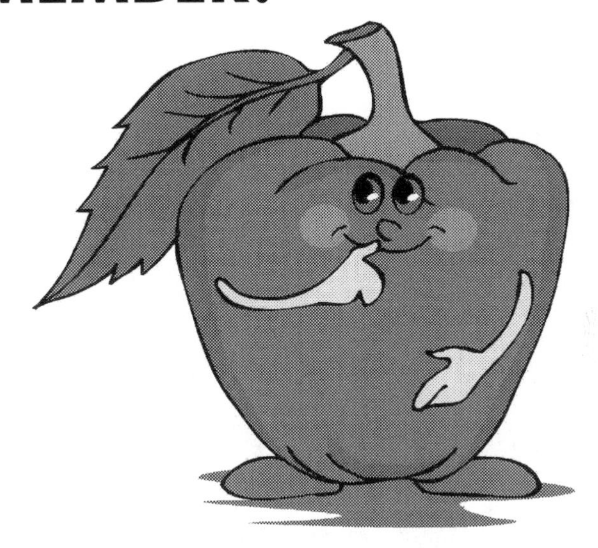

These natural healthy foods will give you a jump-start to a healthier life, and you will look and feel fantastic. You will be amazed at the difference a few changes in your diet can make, and how easy it can be, to a healthier, happier and slimmer you. The results will be undeniably fantastic.

Growing old is a fact of life, but it doesn't have to mean looking tired and feeling lifeless. We know that eating healthy foods will help keep us fit and protect us from disease. Healthy foods can have an effect on how we age. The fact is that good nutritional foods are the cornerstone of looking good and feeling great.

You may be eating plenty of food, but not eating the right foods that give your body the nutrients you need to be healthy. And you may not be getting enough physical activity to stay fit and burn those extra calories. Eating right and being physical active aren't just a diet. Its is the keys to a healthy lifestyle. With these healthful habits, you may reduce your risk of many chronic diseases. So the sooner you start, the better for you, your family, and your future.

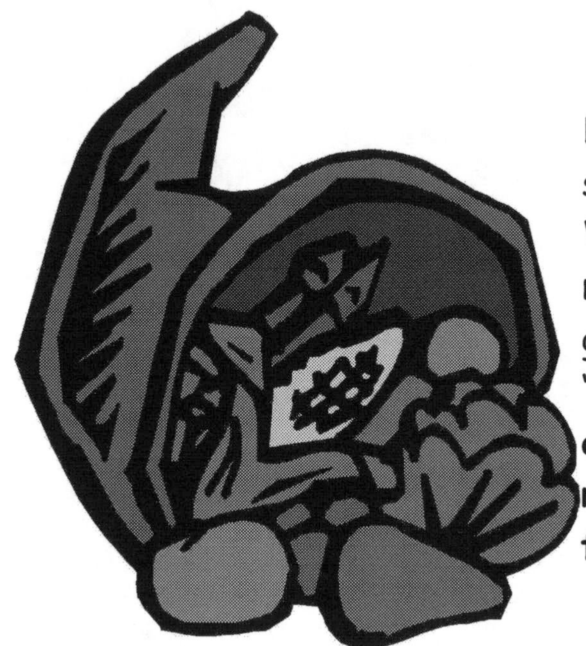

Dietary supplements. Vitamins and minerals are good, **"but there are no replacement for food".**

I have studied nutrition for many years, and Believe you should protect your health by living an active lifestyle. Eating natural foods for vitamin and mineral benefits is also important. Vitamins are essential to sustain life and we must get them from our foods and dietary supplements. Vitamins and minerals are necessary for our growth, vitality and well being. The benefit of vitamins, minerals are many, *"but there are no replacement for food".* A vitamin or mineral has no caloric or energy value by itself. It's important to make smart food choices and watch portion sizes wherever you might be, at work, in your favorite restaurant, or just running errands. Try these tips When grabbing lunch, have a sandwich on whole-grain bread and choose low-fat-free milk, water, or other drink without added sugar. In a restaurant, opt for steamed, grilled, or broiled dishes instead of those that are fried.

Its important to remember that there are six nutrients essential for energy, proper functioning of organs, utilization of food and cell growth: Carbohydrates, proteins, fats, vitamins, minerals and water.

| **PROTEINS** | **CARBOHYDRATES** | **Non-starchy veggies** | **Fruit** |
|---|---|---|---|
| Cheese | Grains | Salads | All fruit |
| Eggs | Pasta | Fresh herbs | |
| Nuts | Rice | Seeds | |
| Fish | Oats | Butter | |
| Game | Bread | Cream | |
| Meat | cookies | Olive oil | |
| Milk | cake | Spices | |
| Poultry | Pastry | | |
| Shellfish | Honey | | |
| Soy products | Maple syrup | | |
| Yogurt | potatoes | | |

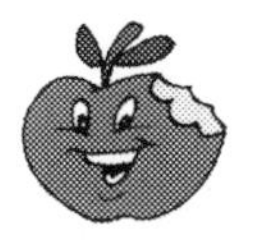

When done correctly, food combining will help your body to burn fat more efficiently, ensure the maximum absorption of nutrients, enzymes and proteins, prevent burping, bloating, gas and indigestion. Without combining the right foods will, make complete digestion impossible, upset digestive enzymes, prevent nutrient uptake. Also you can risk a host of ills, including bloating, heartburn, indigestion, malabsorption, constipation, cramps, irritable bowel syndrome or worse.

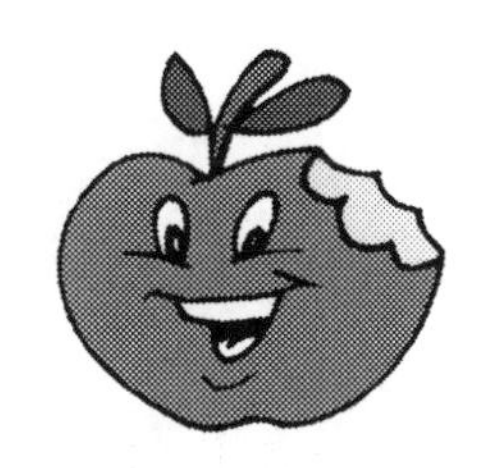

CHAPTER 4

# Vitamins

# VITAMINS

## ( Their Nutritional value)

Vitamins and minerals are recommended daily intakes and are an essential part of you diet. You cannot survive for extended periods of time without.

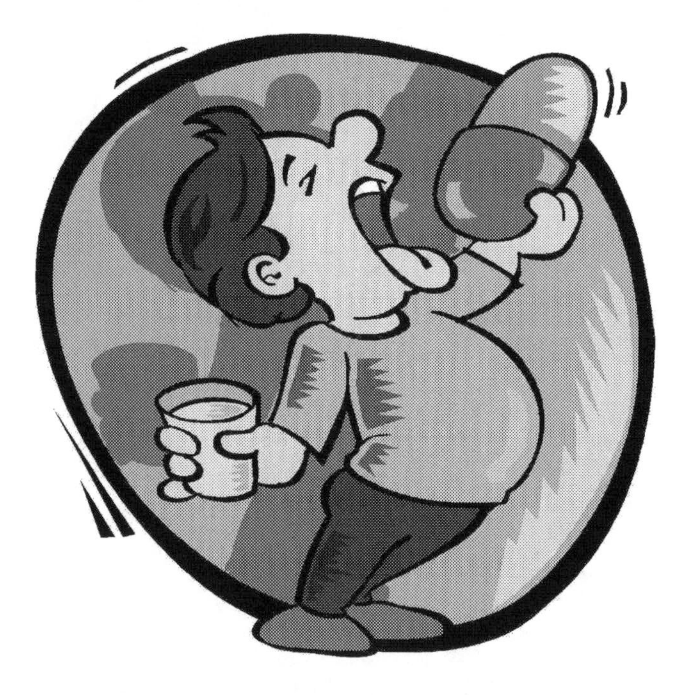

Herbs and phytonutrients can improve your health and well-being, but are not essential. "All vitamins are essential". While minerals generally do not deteriorate vitamins do and their potency diminishes over time. When fruits and vegetables become exposed to sunlight, oxygen an moisture, vitamins will gradually lose potency. Also remember bioavailability refers to the potential a food has to be absorbed into the bloodstream and have the desired affect to maintain a healthy life. So it is important to eat a balance diet of fresh foods.

# Vitamin list below:

**Their benefits in protecting your health.**

**Vitamin A or Retinol:** Eye disorder, acne, skin disorders, infections, healing of wounds.

**Vitamin B1 or Thiamine:** Beriberi, heart diseases, indigestion, body metabolism.

**Vitamin B2 or Riboflavin:** Cataract, skin disorders, body metabolism, immunity, nervous

**Vitamin B3 or Niacin:** Weakness, digestion, nervous system, skin disorders, migraine, blood cholesterol, diabetes, diarrhea

**Vitamin B5 or Pantothenic Acid:** Stress, arthritis, infections, skin disorders,

**Vitamin B6 or Pyridoxamine:** Diabetes, piles, convulsions, excessive menstrual bleeding

**Vitamin B7 or Biotin:** Skin disorders, body metabolism, hair care.

**Vitamin B9 or Folic Acid:** Anemia, digestion, sprue, pregnancy, brain growth skin disorders.

**Vitamin B12 or Cyanocobalamin:** Anemia, smoking, pregnancy, liver disorder, kidney disorder.

**Vitamin C or Ascorbic Acid:** Eye disorders, cancer, scurvy, common cold,infections, high blood pressure, kidney disorder.

**Vitamin D:** Rickets, arthritis, tooth decay, bone repair, immunity, blood circulation, menstrual cycles, eye disorders.

**Vitamin E or Tocopherol:** Anti-aging, skin care, heart diseases, blood circulation, eye disorders.

**Vitamin K:** Internal bleeding, blood clotting, billary obstruction

# Other Key Nutrients

**Antioxidants:** Compound that inhibits the effects of harmful free radicals.

**Free radicals:** Molecules that damage the body's tissues, produced as a by-product of metabolism or environmental factors.

**Gamma-linolenic acid (GLA):** Fatty acid needed for healthy hormone balance, to help lower inflammation and to reduce blood clotting.

**Linoleic acid:** Unsaturated fatty acid considered essential to the human diet.

**Lutein:** Antioxidant carotenoid important for eye health.

**Omega-3-6 fatty acids:** Polyunsaturated fats found in oily fish, nuts and seeds. Studies show that they help to make the blood less liable to clot and so reduce the risk of heart disease.

**Calcium** : For healthy bones, teeth, Muscles, Nerves, and some glands.

**Fiber**: Diets rich in dietary fiber have been shown to have a number of beneficial effects, including decreased risk of coronary heart disease.

**Folate:** With adequate folate may may reduce a women's risk of having a child with a brain or spinal cord defrct.

**Iron:** Needed for healthy blood and normal functioning of all cells.

**Magnesium:** Is necessary for healthy bones and is involved with more than 300 enzymes in your body, inadequate levels may result in muscle cramps and high blood pressure.

**Potassium**: May help to maintain blood pressure.

**Sodium**: For normal cell function in the body.

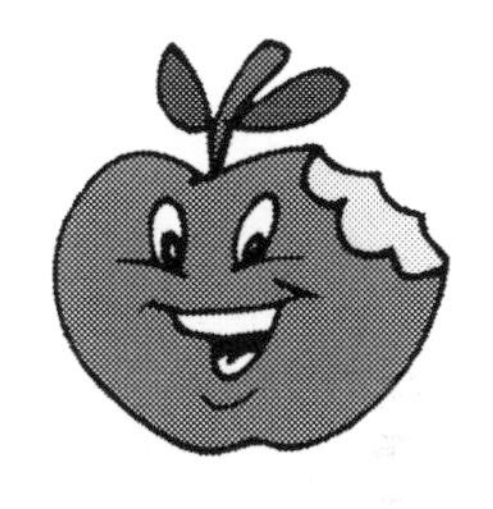

CHAPTER 5

# Ailments

# Ailments:

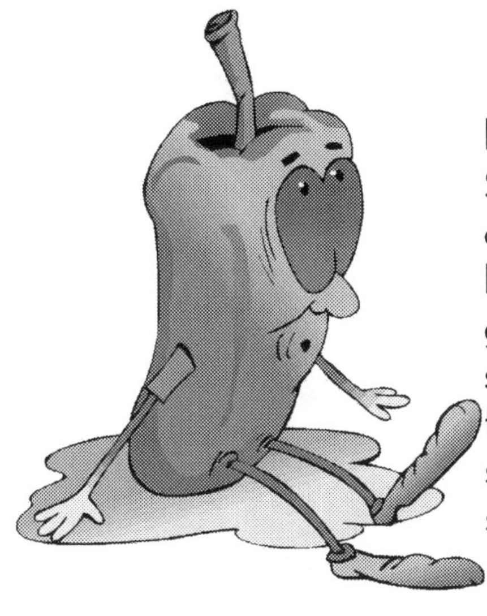

**Foods to eat:**
Spinach, almonds, cashew nut, Lentil, kidney beans, sardine, grains, oats, parsley, seaweed, peaches, flax seeds, sunflower seeds, grapes, yams, squash,

**Fatigue:** If you feel tired all the time, you could be anemic. This condition occurs when there is a decrease in the amount of oxygen-carrying hemoglobin found in your red blood cells. Symptoms include weakness and general fatigue. Eating foods high in iron and vitamin B12 helps to combat anemia at any stage of life. You can change all that. You not be tired any longer. To maximize energy, you need to include certain foods to your diet. Foods that will boost the metabolism and sustain consistent energy levels. The most important nutrients required for energy production are the B complex group of vitamins. Deficiencies in B vitamins can often result in energy slumps. Other metabolism boosting nutrients include vitamin C, magnesium, zinc, iron.

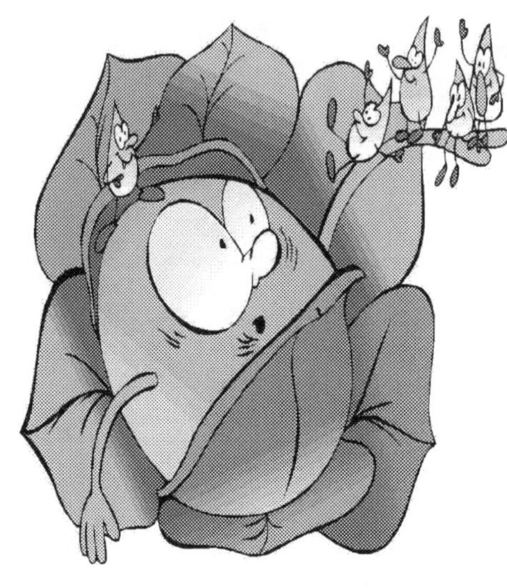

**Foods to eat:**
Grapes, oranges,
prune, spinach,
sweet potato,
almonds, peanuts,
pumpkin seed,
whole wheat,
lentil, kidneys beans,
haddock, oyster,
chicken, parsley,
ginger, coconut oil

**Insomnia:** Sleep quality is key in how you look and feel. Good sleep makes you perform much better both physically and mentally. And helps you to stay healthy and bright. To get a good night's sleep, avoid stimulants such as coffee and chocolate at least five hours before you go to bed. They can cause blood sugar highs and lows. Also when snacking, eat foods containing natural sugars to keep your blood sugar levels stable. Eat your last meal of the day at least a couple of hours before bedtime. When you eat too late, you stress and wear out your body. You cannot digest a late meal effectively if you go to sleep on a full stomach. It is bad for your digestive organs, heart and liver.

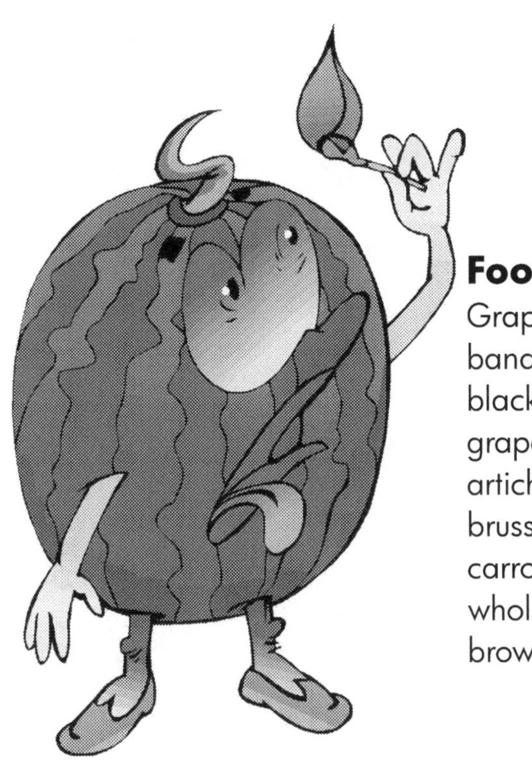

**Foods to eat:**
Grapes, papaya,
banana,
black currants,
grapefruit, watercress,
artichoke,
brussels sprout,
carrots, almonds,
whole wheat,
brown rice

**Digestive Problems:** Digestive problems, such as heart burn don't have to be an inevitable aspect of getting old. Keeping the digestive system in good shape is to eat plenty of fiber-rich foods and drink plenty of water. If you suffer from indigestion discomfort and a burning feeling. Try to reduce your intake of acid forming foods, such as red meat and cheese and eat more foods containing digestive enzymes and fiber. Chewing slowly until food becomes liquefied is important. Really savor each bite, feel the texture and capture the flavor of your food. It is when you saliva comes into contact with your food, as being chewed, that the digestive process begins. The chewed food will then pass easily through your digestive system with maximum nutrient uptake. Digestive problems are usually caused by heavy consumption of greasy or spicy foods or eating to much to fast.

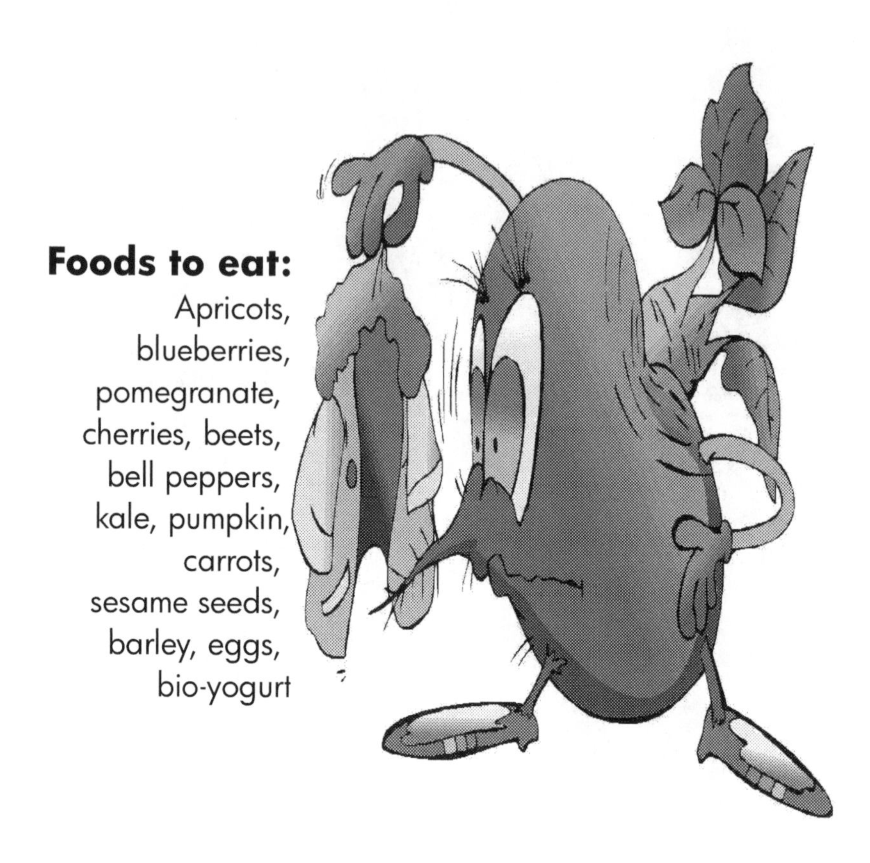

**Foods to eat:**
Apricots, blueberries, pomegranate, cherries, beets, bell peppers, kale, pumpkin, carrots, sesame seeds, barley, eggs, bio-yogurt

**Eye Disease:** If you want to keep your eyes in great condition, remember the old adage about eating your carrots. In fact, any brightly colored fruit and vegetable. Studies suggest that the antioxidants they contain including vitamins A, C, and E and lutein benefit the eyes by helping the lenses adjust to changes in light; maintaining the macula. The part of the eye that enables clear vision. Also keep the eyes moist.

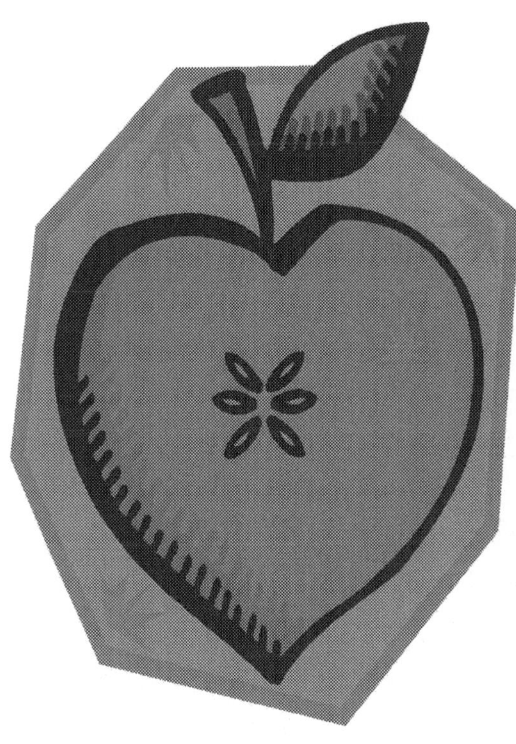

**Food to eat:**
Grapes, papaya,
cranberries,
Cantaloupes, melon,
grapefruit,
pomegranate,
avocado, bell peppers,
onions, broccoli,
Cabbage, mushroom,
asparagus, almonds,
flax seeds, oats,
barley, soybean,
sardine,
green tea, garlic,
fennel, coconut

**Heart Disease:** You can go a long way by avoiding foods containing saturated fats, which raise your cholesterol levels and can clog your arteries. Make sure you use healthy mono saturated oils and eat foods containing flavonoids and plenty of fiber. Avoid foods that may be saturated, polyunsaturated or monounsaturated these are raised by excess intake of fat and alcohol. Regular cardiovascular exercise, can go a long way.

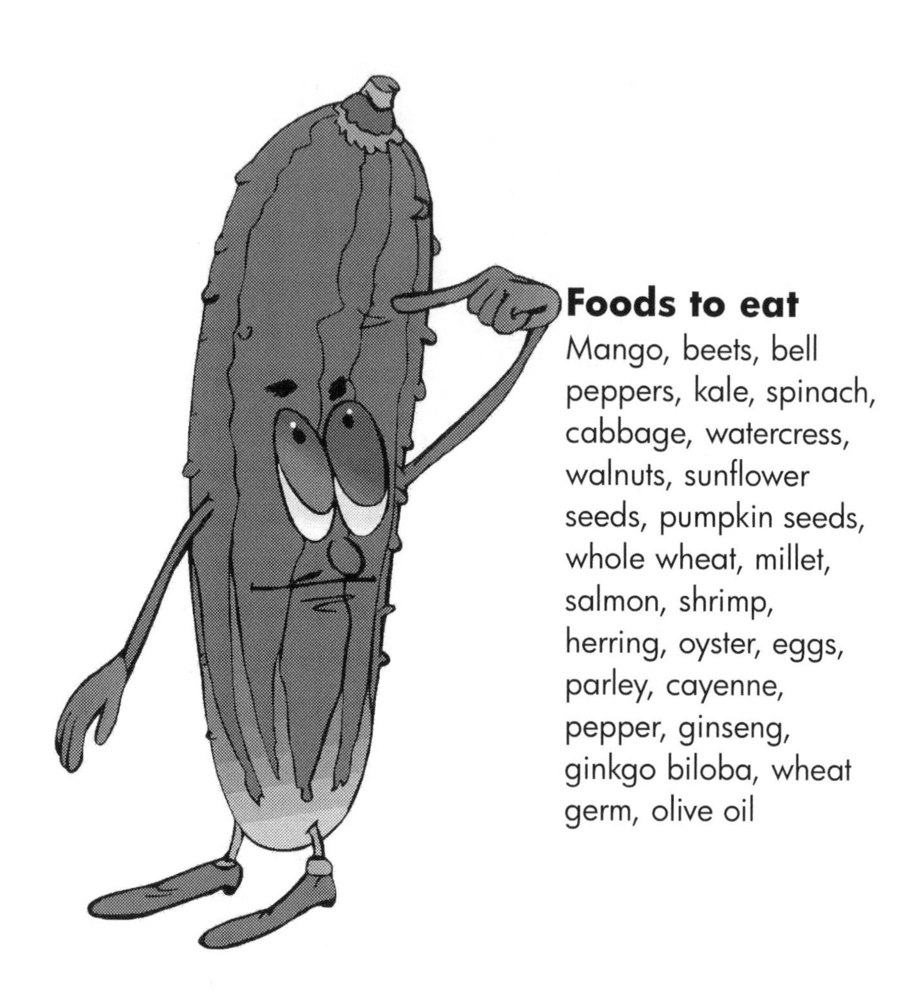

**Foods to eat**

Mango, beets, bell peppers, kale, spinach, cabbage, watercress, walnuts, sunflower seeds, pumpkin seeds, whole wheat, millet, salmon, shrimp, herring, oyster, eggs, parley, cayenne, pepper, ginseng, ginkgo biloba, wheat germ, olive oil

**Memory Loss:** Researchers are studying the possibility that foods high in antioxidants particularly vitamins C and E and the mineral silica, this may help to keep our brains fit and active in later years. As we get older our bodies start to make less chemicals the brain cells need to work, thus making it harder to recall stored information.

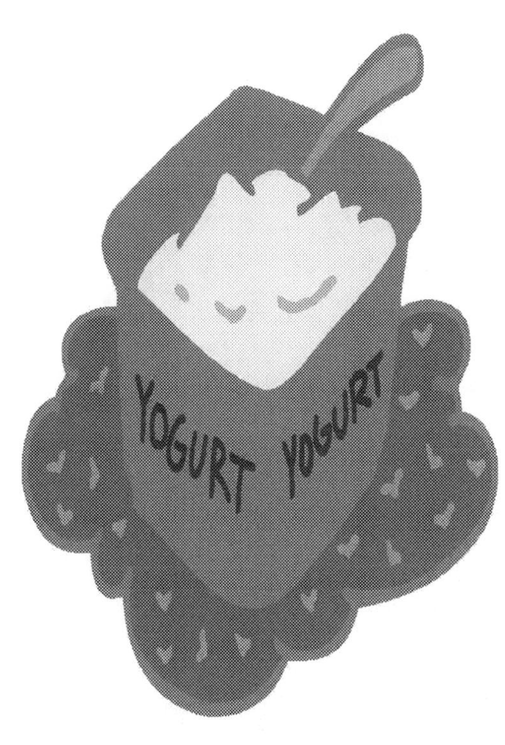


**Foods to eat:**
Cucumber, Broccoli,
spinach,
pumpkin seeds,
flax seeds,
herring, haddock,
oyster, milk,
yogurt, parsley,
ginger, soy,
cayenne pepper,
olive oil,
sesame seeds

**Osteoporosis:** A diet rich in calcium is critical for maintaining bone strength throughout life. Vitamin D is also important, as it helps the body to absorb calcium. Bone lost occurs as you age, and unless we take the precautions, you can find yourself suffering from osteoporosis. Calcium can be obtained from sesame seeds, dark leafy green vegetables, soy foods and yogurt. Although milk or dairy products contain significant amounts of calcium, they are insufficiently assimilated by the body and it is best to replace with plant sources. Magnesium, silica and other vital minerals for bones are found in most vegetables and whole grains.

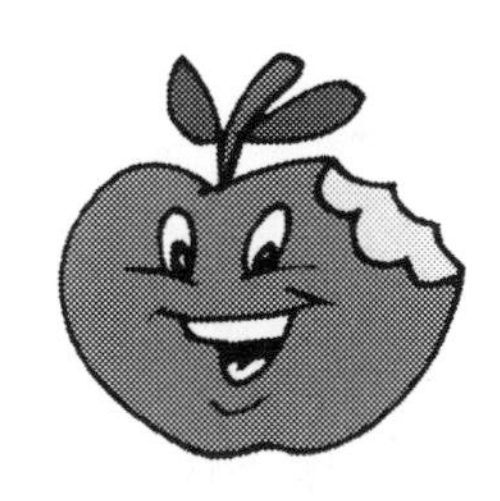

CHAPTER 6

# Remedies

## Remedies, discover the power of food

**Allergy** – Onion

**Anemia** – Apricot, Beans, beets,, Cantaloupe, Celery, Cherries, Corn, Dates, Grapes, Kelp, Lettuce

**Anorexia** – Lettuce, Radish

**Antihelmintic –** Apple, Apricot, Bamboo shoots, Cherries, Coconut Meat, Onion, Papaya seeds, Peach, Pepper (hot), Pineapple, Pumpkin seeds, Sesame seeds, Squash seeds, water, Chestnuts, Watermelon seeds.

**Arthritis and Rheumatism** – Apple, Cabbage, Cantaloupe, Cauliflower, Celery, Cherries, Corn, Cucumber, Grape, Grapefruit, Lettuce, Lime, Mustard greens, Orange, Pepper (green) , Pineapple, Strawberries, Tangerine.

**Asthma** – Apricot, Cauliflower, Celery, Cherries, Guava, Onion, Orange, Peach, pepper (hot), Tangerine.

**Blood purifier** – Cabbage, Cauliflower.

**Blood Hyperacidity** – Celery, Grape, Guava, Mango, Mustard (greens), Peach, Pear, Pepper (green).

**Brain development** – Kelp, Celery, Soybean, Fish (omega-3)

**Cancer** – Apple, Apricot, Asparagus, Beets, Broccoli, Cantaloupe, Carrot, Cauliflower, Cherries, Corn, Lettuce, Mustard, Okra, Papaya, Peach, Peas, Pepper (green) Potato (sweet), Prunes, Pumpkin, Spinach, Squash, Tangerine, Tomato, Watermelon.

**Cramps** – Cherries.

## Remedies, discover the power of food

**Diarrhea –** Apple, Banana, Beets.

**Deafness** – Cabbage.

**Diabetes** – Alfalfa, Celery, Cucumber, Onion, Radish, Soybean, Spinach.

**Diaper rash** – Corn starch, Lecithin (liquid).

**Dizziness** – Onion.

**Diuretic** – Celery, Cucumber, Onion, Pumpkin, Pumpkin seeds, Radish, Tamarind, Watermelon.

**Eyes** – Cabbage, Carrot, Onion.

**Gall-Bladder** – Apricot, Radish, Soybean, Tomato.

**Goiter** – Coconut, Kelp, Pineapple.

**Hair Growth** – Cabbage, Carrot, Cucumber, Lettuce, Onion, Radish, Rice (brown) Spinach.

If you start eating all these different natural foods you have read about in the pages of this book. I will assure you that you will be doing a great service to your body. And general overall health.

As you can see after reading this information, there is an abundance of many healthy natural foods that you may or may not have been eating. Now its time to introduce these foods to your diet and start living life to the fullest.

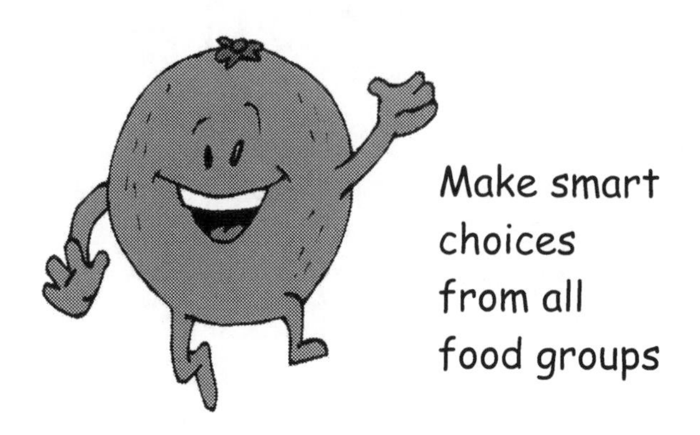

## Make smart choices from all food groups

The best way to give your body the balanced nutrition it needs is by eating a variety of nutrient packed foods every day. Just be sure to stay within your daily calorie needs. A healthy eating plan is one that emphasizes fruits, vegetables, whole grains, and low fat or fat free dairy products. Include lean meats, poultry, fish, beans, eggs, and nuts. Stay away from saturated fats, trans-fats, cholesterol, salt and added sugars.

Drink plenty of water at least 6-8 glasses a day, though you might need more water during hot weather and when exercising. Adequate water is essential for keeping your skin hydrated and for eliminating toxins through the kidneys and colon.

Also make sure you include lots of fiber in your diet. It keeps your intestinal tract regular, and enhances the elimination of waste products from your body.

Also make sure your diet contains plenty of antioxidants, which help slow down cellular aging. Fresh fruits and vegetables are the best sources of natural plant antioxidants.

By eating protein and carbohydrates at separate meals, you can prevent unnecessary fermentation in the colon and increase nutrient absorption into the blood.

## Heart - Healthy Eating

Your total intake of saturated fat should not exceed 18 grams. Follow these guidelines to help you meet the American Heart Association's recommendations, which include limiting your fat intake to 30 percent or less of total calories and limit your saturated fat intake to 10 percent or less of total calories.

| Total Calories | Total from fat | Total Fat (gm) | Total Saturate Fat (gm) |
|---|---|---|---|
| 1,600 | 480 | 53 | 18 |
| 2,000 | 600 | 67 | 22 |
| 2,200 | 660 | 73 | 24 |
| 2,500 | 750 | 83 | 28 |
| 2,800 | 840 | 93 | 31 |
| 3,200 | 960 | 107 | 35 |

## Blood Lipid Levels

| LIPID | DESIRABLE LEVELS |
|---|---|
| Total Blood Cholesterol | <200 mg/dL |
| LDL Cholesterol | <130 mg/dL |
| HDL Cholesterol | >35 mg/dL |
| Blood Triglycerides | <250 mg/dL |

Two sources of cholesterol, one source is made by the body and the other from foods of animal origin only, such as meat, fish, and dairy foods; These can be decreased by low cholesterol/low-fat diet, high-fiber diet, exercise, weight loss, controlled blood pressure and controlled diabetes.

**LDL Cholesterol –** Low-Density Lipoproteins, **Bad** blood cholesterol, stays in the arteries so it can build up. You can decease by low-fat diet, fiber diet, weight loss and exercise.

**HDL Cholesterol –** High-Density Lipoproteins, **Good** blood cholesterol, helps in the removal from arteries. You can increase by exercise, weight loss, and low-fat diet.

**Monounsaturated Fats –** MUFA: lowers blood cholesterol levels and raises HDL cholesterol; found in olive oil, peanut oil and some fish.

**Polyunsaturated Fats –** Lowers blood cholesterol levels; found in corn oil, soybean oil, sunflower oil and some fish.

**Saturated Fats –** Raises blood cholesterol levels; found in all animal products and vegetable oils, such as stick margarine, butter, coconut oil and palm oil.

**Triglycerides –** From of fat in food; may be saturated, polyunsaturated or monounsaturated, these are raised by excess intake of fat and alcohol; You can decease by low-fat diet, weight loss, exercise and alcohol in moderation.

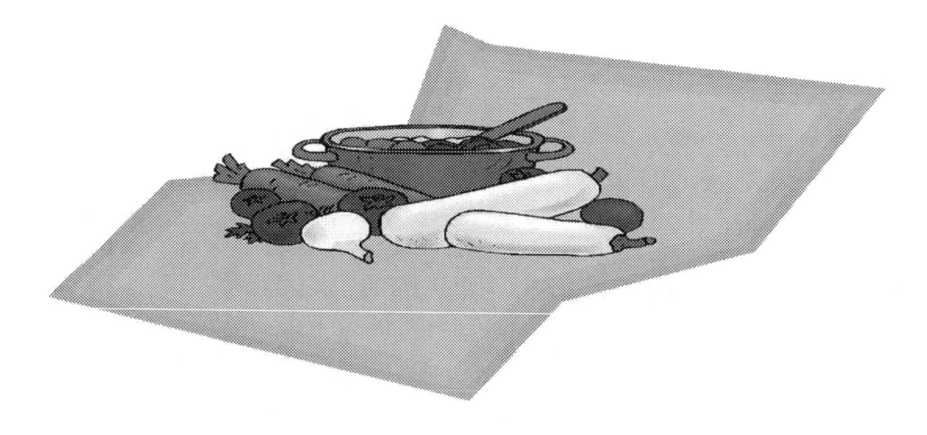

# Support the Liver

Eating the right healthy foods is crucial, to keep the liver healthy. Since the liver must process the by-products of what we eat. To make the job easier eat unprocessed foods as much as possible. Prepackaged foods are loaded with chemicals, preservatives, colorings and flavorings overwork the liver. Foods such as Cake, cookies, processed, refined or fired foods lack nutrients and are improperly absorbed, further weakening the liver. Eat more of the following healthy foods, which are specifically nourishing to the liver function.

## Fruits, Grains, Legumes, Vegetables

At times of stress or when you are just tired it is easy to reach for a quick sugar fix, like cookies, cake, ice cream, chocolate. Train yourself to indulge in some of the following foods.

**Fresh fruits** help to stimulate energy flow through the liver, especially dark grapes, blackberries, blueberries, raspberries and strawberries. It is better to eat fruit by itself.

**Grains,** such as amaranth, millet, quinoa.

**Vegetables,** such as asparagus, basil, bay leaves, beets, black pepper, celery, cucumber, radish, dill, fennel, garlic.

**Legumes,** Kidney beans, peas, soybeans.

**Other foods,** such as Ginger, Lemon, Mustard greens, onions, beets, radish, romaine lettuce, rosemary, watercress.

**Foods containing sulfur,** These vegetables are full of an specific liver building enzymes. Broccoli, nuts, brussels sprouts, cabbage, cauliflower, flax, sunflower, pumpkin seeds.

# Skin care

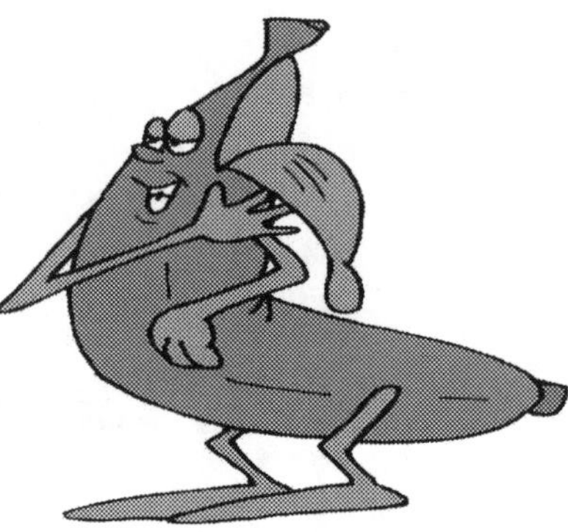

Most people don't think about the skin being an organ, but it is the largest organ in your body. It accounts for approximately 16 percent of your body weight. It also protects delicate internal structures, also assists in colon, lungs and kidneys in the elimination of toxic waste. There many factors that affect the health of your skin, these include heredity, age, climate, pollution, diet, stress and fluctuations in hormones. Changes in your complexion is caused by these two factors. How well your internal eliminator organs are working and weather or not your body is lacking in vitamins and minerals. And both of these factor, in turn, influence each other.

**Drink** plenty of clean water, at least 6-8 glasses per day. Adequate water is essential for keeping the skin hydrated and for eliminating toxins through the kidneys and colon.

**Include** fiber in your diet, it keeps your intestinal tract regular, and enhances the elimination of waste products from your body.

**Make** sure your diet contains plenty of antioxidants. Will help slow down cellular aging. Fresh fruits and vegetables are the best sources of natural plant antioxidants.

**Bad fats** are detrimental to your body, essential fatty acids (good fats) are vital for healthy skin. You can obtain these from dark leafy green vegetables, whole grains, seeds, nuts, soybeans, cold pressed oils, especially flax, pumpkin, sunflower, sesame and oily fish such as sardines, mackerel and wild salmon.

**Reduce** foods that clog, the worst offenders are red meat, dairy, refined foods, fried foods and foods that contain hydrogenated oils or fats

# STRESS

**A well balanced diet is crucial in preserving health and helping to reduce stress.**

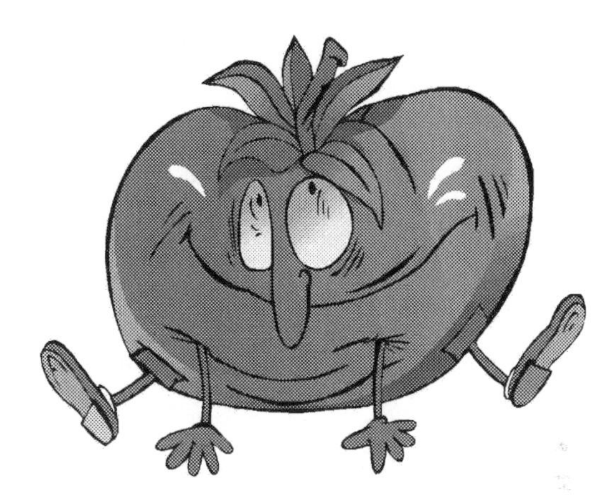

Certain foods and drinks act as powerful stimulants to the body and are a direct cause of stress. The stimulation, although quite pleasurable in the short term, can be quite harmful in the long term.

**FOODS TO AVOID**

**Caffeine** this is found in coffee, tea, chocolate, coke, etc. It causes the release of adrenaline, thus increasing the level of stress. There is suggested that there is a link between caffeine intake and high blood pressure and high cholesterol levels.

**Alcohol** like caffeine, taken in moderation, alcohol is useful drug. It has been shown in studies to benefit cardiovascular system. Alcohol is a major cause of stress. The irony of the situation is that most people take to drinking as a way to combat stress, but in actuality, they make it worse by consuming alcohol.

**Salt** increases blood pressure, deplete adrenal glands, and causes emotional instability.

**Fat** avoid the consumption of foods high in saturated fats. Fats cause obesity and out unnecessary stress on the cardiovascular system.

**Sugar** has no essential nutrients. It provides a short-term boost of energy through the body, resulting possibly in the exhaustion of the adrenal glands. This can result in irritability, poor concentration and depression.

# FOODS TO EAT

Whole grains promote the production of brain neurotransmitter serotonin, which increases your sense of well-being. Also green, orange and yellow vegetables are high in minerals, vitamins and phytochemicals, which boost immune response and protect against disease.

**Carbohydrates** trigger release of the brain neurotransmitter serotonin, which soothes you. Studies suggest that the carbohydrates present in a baked potato, spaghetti or rice, is enough to relieve the anxiety of a stressful day.

**Fiber** eat more fiber to keep your digestive system moving. Stress result in cramps and constipation. Your meals should provide at least 25 grams of fiber per day. Fruits, vegetables and grains are excellent sources of fiber.

**Vegetables** your brain production of serotonin, is sensitive to your diet. Eating more vegetables, can increase your brain's serotonin production. This increase is due to improved absorption of the amino acid L-Tryptophan. Vegetables contain the natural, safe, from of L-Tryptophan. Meats contain natural L-Tryptophan also, but when you eat meat, the L-tryptophan has to compete with so many other amino acids for absorption that the L-Tryptonphan lose out. The result is that you get better absorption of L-Tryptonphan when eating vegetables.

NOTE: The information in this book is not intended as a substitute for medical treatment and advice. It is advisable to consult a medical professional before using any of these methods. Particularly if you or suffering from a medical condition and are unsure of the suitability of any of the remedies of foods mentioned in this book. A dietitian or doctor should be consulted before any change in diet.

# TEETH & GUMS

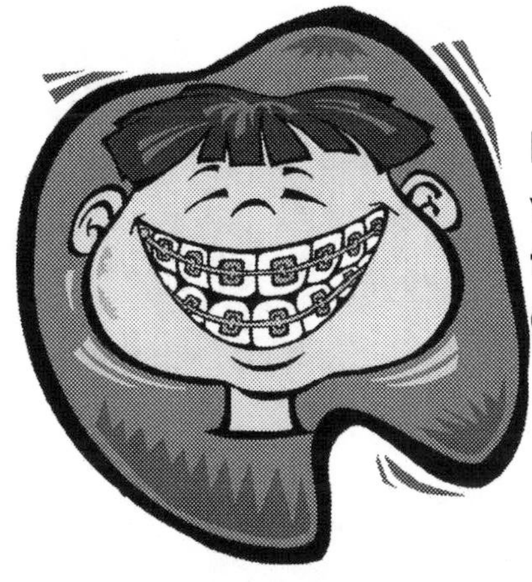

**Keep that smile, with good teeth and gum care.**

**First and foremost** it is important to bush your teeth after very meal. Also it is important to eat the right foods to prevent an imbalances of mineral deficiencies and poor dental hygiene, this will make gums susceptible to bleeding. Poor hygiene will also put your teeth under strain. Teeth need the same nutrition as your bones to stay healthy , strong and of course pearly white. Although there is an significant amount of calcium in milk and dairy products. It is not insufficiently assimilated by the body. Vegetables can give you a better source of calcium through green leafy vegetables, soy products, magnesium, silica and other vital minerals for your teeth are found in most whole grains and vegetables.

# Children, health and well-being

**Be sure that your children get at least 60 minutes of physical actively a day**

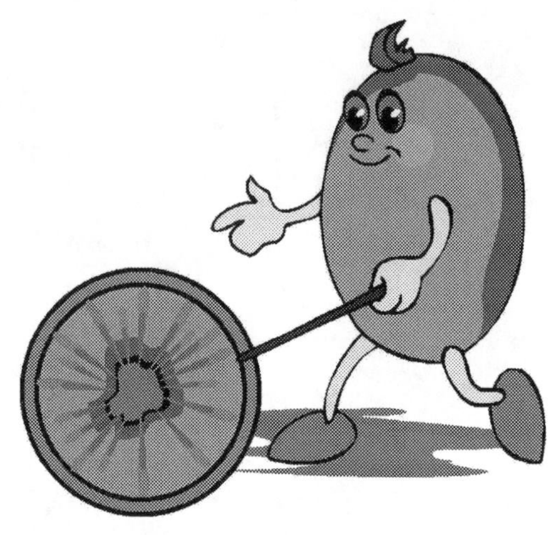

It is important that your children stay physically active, to maintain good health. The body is designed to move and stay active. And for children it is very important because they are in the stage of development, and to keep their muscles toned they need to have fun physical activities.

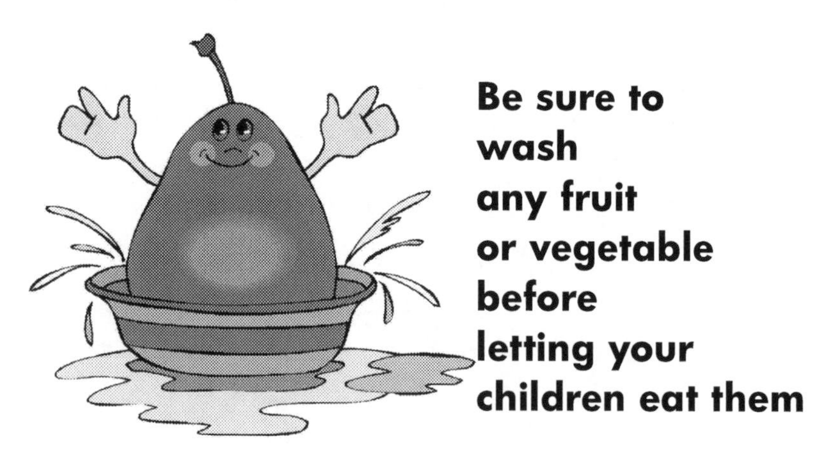

**Be sure to wash any fruit or vegetable before letting your children eat them**

It is also very important to have a good balance diet of good natural foods. This will give your children a good and healthy life. Brain development, healthy teeth and bones and overall well-being.

The greatest gift you can give your children, love, guidance, support, and be sure they get the nutrients they need to have a full healthy life. It is so important for them to have all the food groups on a daily bases.

Use the food pyramid, as a guide. At the base of the health food pyramid includes all plants foods, vegetables, fruits, nuts, beans, lentils and grain cereals, bread (preferably wholegrain) These foods contain many different nutrients and should make up most of the food they eat.

At the middle of the pyramid, include fish, lean meat, eggs, chicken, milk, cheese, and yogurt. These foods should be eaten in moderation. They should have 4 to 6 servings in the first section and 1 to 2 serving in the second section. These foods should help provide protein, minerals, (especially iron and calcium) and B vitamins. Alongside encourage water consumption. 6 – 8 glasses each day is the recommendation. Smaller children about 4 – 5 glasses of water.

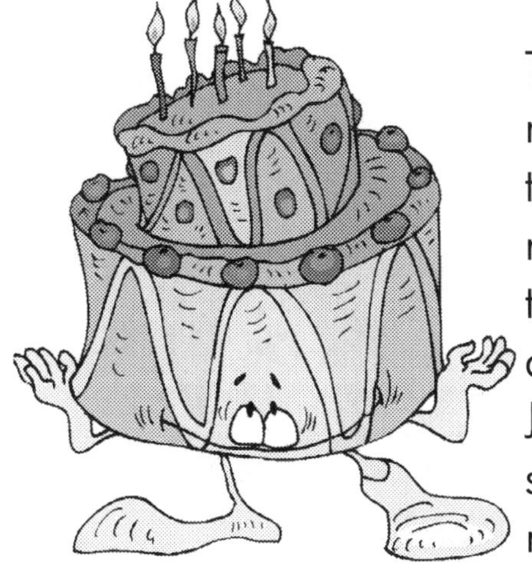

This does not mean they can not have a occasional treat once in a while. Just make sure it is moderation.

# EXERCISE

I'm talking
about simple,
gentle movement.
The type that
will keep the
body toned

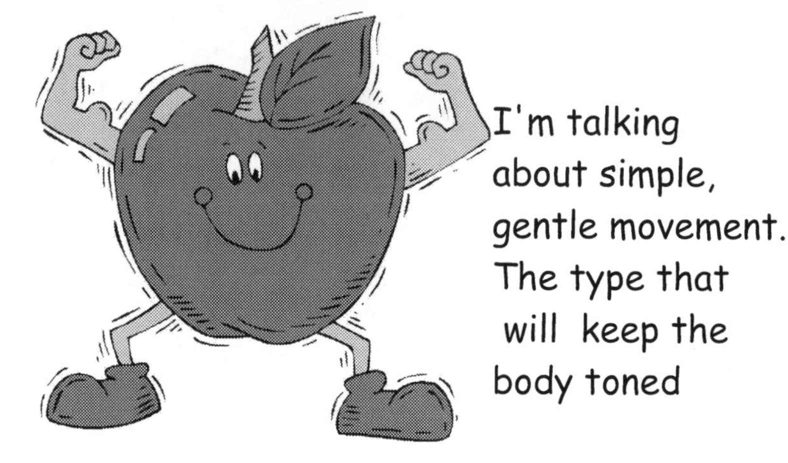

**Find your balance between food and physical activity**

Consider this, if you eat 100 more food calories a day than you burn, you will gain around a pound a month. That's about 10 or more pounds in a year. The fact is to lose weight, it's important to reduce calories and increase physical activity. In order to properly keep your body in tip-top shape, its essential to exercise. This does not mean you need to embark upon a vigorous body building plan that you will need to go to the gym on a daily basis. Just do some stretching exercise, a nice walk, step-climbing, swimming and even dancing or any other moderate fun movements would be excellent if done on a regular basis. These exercises should last at least thirty to sixty minutes a day. But any thing you can do that will make you break into a sweat is even better. These are just a few things you can do to keep your body fit. Exercise will also help in detoxifying your body, so drink water it is the most efficient detoxifying fluids we can give ourselves each day. I would recommend 6-8 glasses of water a day. Children and teenagers should be physically active for 60 minutes every day, or most every day.

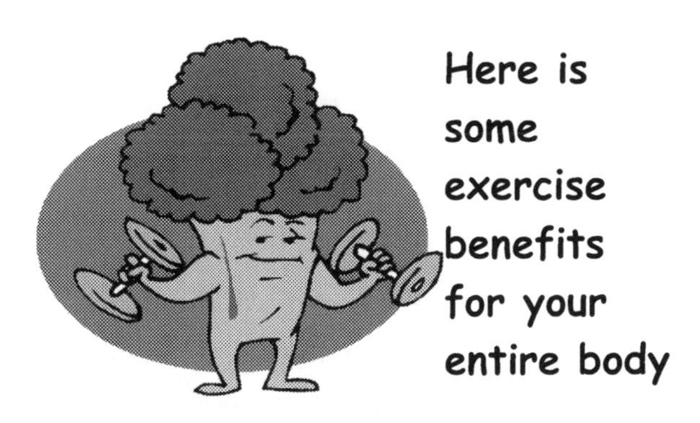

## Here is some exercise benefits for your entire body

If you have not been exercising regularly, check with your doctor before beginning any new program. If you have such things like high blood pressure or other risk factors for heart disease, work with your doctor to determine a safe and effective exercise plan. Begin your exercise regimen slowly and have plenty of patience. Don't over do it at first. Trying to do to much too fast could lead to muscle strain, back problems, or any other number of joint or muscle disorders.

There are many reason to begin and/or maintain a regular exercise program. Improving your physical activity level may lower your blood pressure, and also help prevent heart attacks and strokes. Numerous studies and research have shown that an active lifestyle prolongs and improves the quality of life. These have been shown to lower blood pressure, aerobic exercise, such as walking, jogging or riding a bike. Something as simple as a regular walking program, such as 30 to 60 minutes, three to four times weekly, can improve your circulation and breathing, while at the same time conditioning your body. Some other cardiovascular fitness actives include hiking, swimming; and participating in aerobics classes and sports such as basketball, racquetball and tennis. If it's to hot to exercise outdoors, find an indoor facility or work out early in the morning to avoid the hottest part of the day. Avoid dehydration by drinking plenty of water before, during and after exercising.

# Overview

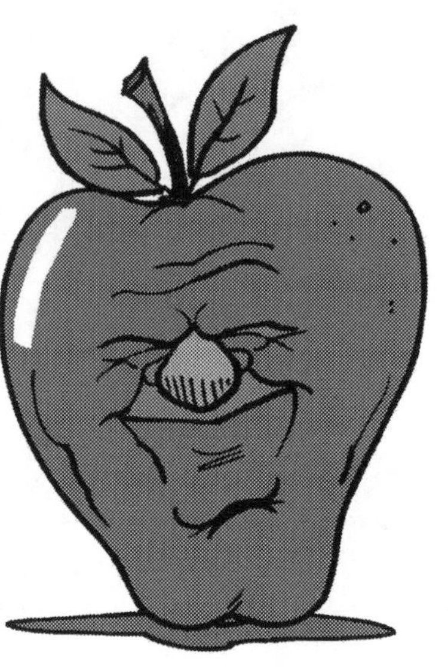

It is inevitable that we are going to grow old, it is just a FACT OF LIFE. It dose not mean we need to look tired and feel lifeless. So you should eat nutritional healthy foods, and exercise it will keep you feeling fit and protect you from disease. The fact is that eating nutritional healthy foods can have an effect on how you age. Choosing the right foods can slow down many signs of aging. And can be a powerful weapon in the battle against health problems such as heart disease, eye conditions, osteoporosis, arthritis and high blood pressure. Also these natural nutritional foods can help keep you fit, strengthen your immune system, increase your resistances to colds and other infections, boosting your energy levels, and improving physical and mental performance.

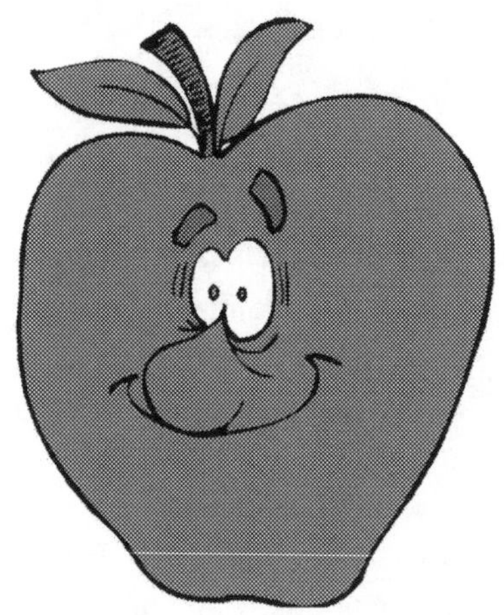

Now is the time to invest in your future health. If you want to stay fit, feel great, look younger and live longer. Than use these facts that you have read in these pages, this information will give you a great start to a long incredible life.

Lets review what you have learned in the previous pages, about your health and eating the right natural foods. The body has trillions of cells, each one demands a constant supply of daily nutrients in order to function. Food affects all those cells, and by extension every aspect of your being, energy levels, thinking, sleeping habits, mood, food cravings, sex drive, and your over all health.

Foods we eat are like fuel, it gives our bodies the energy to function well. If you don't make good food choices (fuel for your body) it can effect your well being, you just won't feel as healthy as you could. The relationship between natural healthy food and your health is significant. Diet plays a vital part in promoting good health and well being.

To get the most from your diet, it is vital to choose natural food with integrity, fresh, natural and unadulterated produce is a powerful source of life enhancing nutrients. These give the body the necessary means to stay healthy and function efficiently. Which will help you feel fit and look younger.

Remember these crucial steps to make the connection between "good food" choices and great health, and "poor food" choices and poor health. Eating natural healthy foods is the key to your well being.

## BAD FOOD FACTS

Studies have shown, on average it is estimated, a third of cancers could be prevented by changes in your diet. One that is high in fiber and whole grains and low in fat. This diet has the potential to prevent a number of cancers, including breast, colon, stomach cancer. Also a diet high in fat, sugar and salt can lead to weight gain and a risk of obesity, heart disease, diabetes, cancer and even infertility. Also associated with fatigue, poor physical and mental performance.

**A diet high in saturated fat and high in salt is associated with an increased risk of heart disease.**

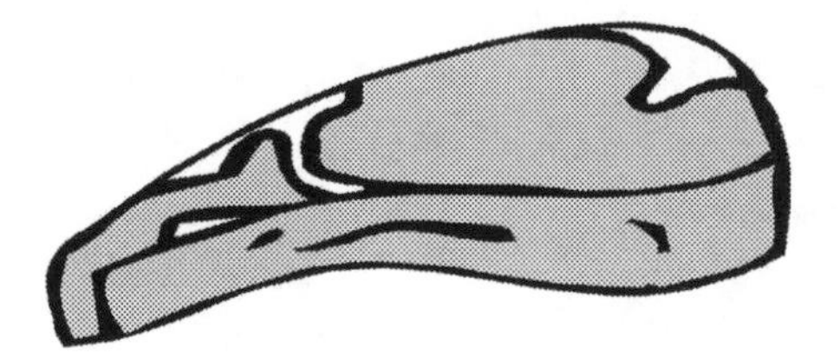

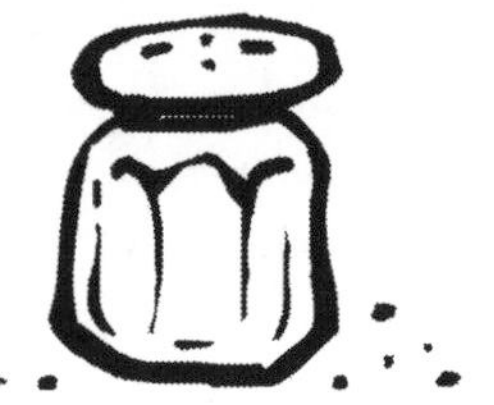

If your diet is poor it can compromise the immune system, this can make you more susceptible to colds, flu and over all poor health. You need a steady balanced of essential vitamins and minerals to keep the immune system working properly, this will provide the protection from infections and disease.

## THE GOOD FOODS

Whole raw foods: These foods have not been cooked, boiled, stewed, microwaved, frozen, baked or steamed. The result, they are still in their original natural state and contain all the natural enzymes. These enzymes are the life force of food which helps the digestion process. Raw vegetables, fruit, whole grains and seeds all contain food enzymes. We need an abundant supply of these enzymes to nourish our bodies, balance our metabolism and provide us with energy. Unprocessed foods are foods that have not had added chemicals or any other additives. These foods are still in their original state, the way nature grew them.

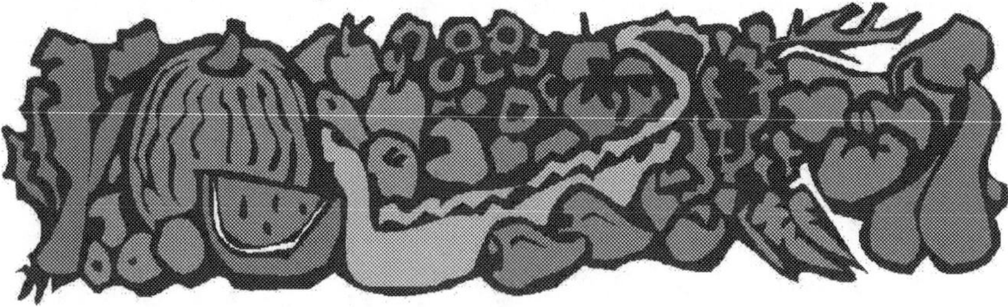

## The Author George Edward Weigel

Is the founder of Cedar Creek Research (development, processing and marketing of agricultural products) and a freelance writer specializing in healthy natural nutritional foods and exercise. George has studied nutrition for many years. Believes you should protect your health by living an active lifestyle. Also we should fuel our bodies with natural nutritional foods from mother earth. Realizing the demand of the bodies trillions of cells, their need of a constant supply of daily nutrients in order to function. It only makes sense the fresher and the more natural our food, the better it will be for overall health. If you don't fuel you body with the right quality or quantity, you won't feel as healthy as you could and should. Healthy eating is the key to our well-being. George is also the author of **"The Blue Barn"** a how to book on the benefit of self-sustaining organic gardening. Believes there is noting like or better than fresh fruits and vegetables right out of the garden. George has done years of research on organic gardening, organic compost, organic soil preparation and research on animal feeds etc. George believes in sustainable agriculture, which focuses on high outputs without depleting the earth's resources or polluting its environment. A strategy to incorporate organic, natural and biodiversity concepts without using any dangerous chemicals, and a source of natural harmony with nature.

## ALSO AVAILABLE:

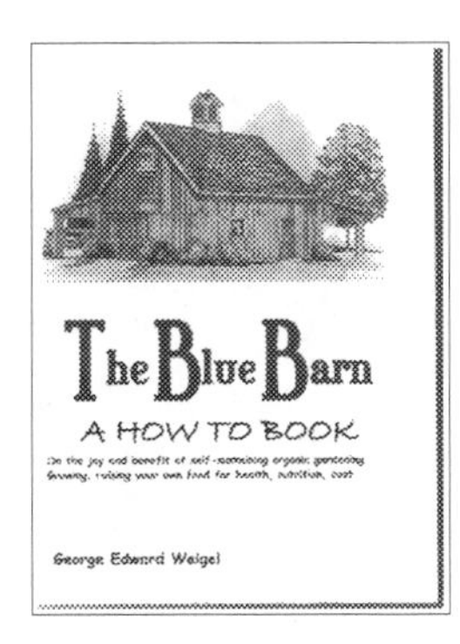


**The Blue Barn**

A How To Book

On the joy and benefit of self-sustaining organic gardening

# CONCLUSION

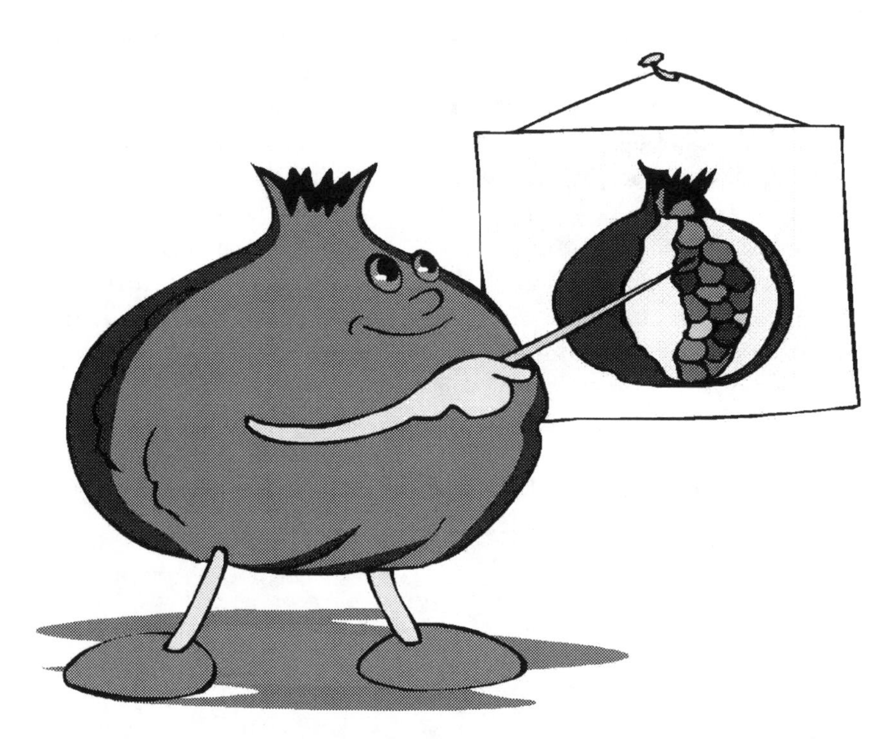

You now know, how, why, the importance of healthy eating. I hope that within these pages of "***An-Apple-A-Day***" I have given you new ideas, new foods, new lifestyle and send you on your way to an amazing healthy body and overall great health for your well-being. Once you understand the powerful nature of energy, from natural foods you will appreciate the impact of this advice. The bottom line is that in order to achieve great health, stay youthful and have a fantastic body, it is important to eat the right natural foods. Eating natural foods for their vitamin and mineral benefits is also important. Vitamins are essential to sustain life and we must get them from our foods and dietary supplements.

## The benefit of vitamins and minerals

Are many, but there is no replacement for natural foods. Vitamins or mineral have no caloric or energy value by itself. Vitamins and minerals are necessary for our growth, vitality and well being. It is important to remember that there are six nutrients essential for energy, proper functioning of organs, utilization of food and cell growth. They are **Carbohydrates, Protein, Fats, Vitamins, Minerals, Water.**

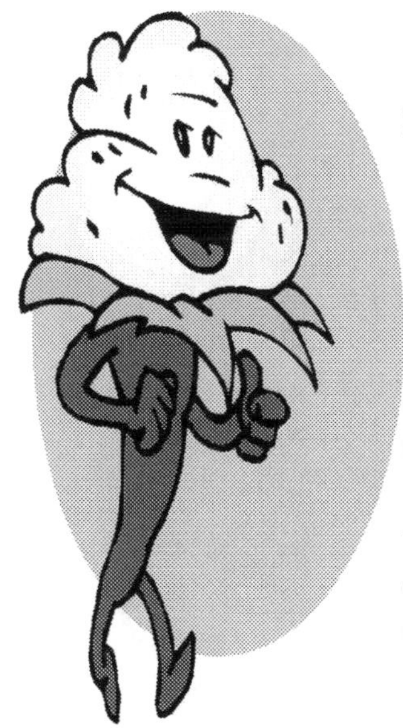

Take a nice walk, it will be great for your heart health!

**Lets not forget exercise,** even if you eat all the right foods, you will still need to do some kind of physical exercise to keep your body toned and fit. Once again there are many reasons to begin or maintain regular exercise program. First, an improved physical activity level may lower your blood pressure, and prevent heart attacks and strokes. Numerous studies and research have shown that an active lifestyle prolongs and improves the quality of life. Such as aerobic exercise, walking, jogging or riding a bike. It is wise to read up on the sport or activity you have chosen, before starting. Also it is important if you have not been exercising regularly, to check with your doctor before beginning any program. Begin your exercise regimen slowly and have plenty of patience. Don't overdo it, trying to do to much too fast could lead to muscle strain, back problems and joint disorders. Remember exercise benefits your entire body. The sooner you start, the better for you, your family, and your future.

It will take some will power at first for some people, but a good diet can prevent illness, combat stress, and leave you looking great. It has long been established that a good healthy diet, eating natural nutritional foods is the cornerstone of a long life. The great thing is that eating good food is one of life's greatest pleasures.

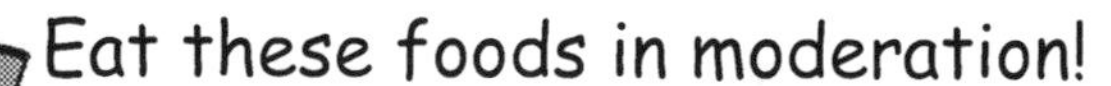

## Eat these foods in moderation!

For some of you, this dose not mean totally cutting out on foods, like barbecues, cake, a little ice cream, etc. These should be in moderation and occasional treats. If you do eat some barbecue meat, make sure that you have some fresh fruit and/or vegetables to go along with it. The antioxidants will help fight off the free-radicals from smoked meats.

## Also if you are going to enjoy a beer with your barbecue, make it a lite beer.

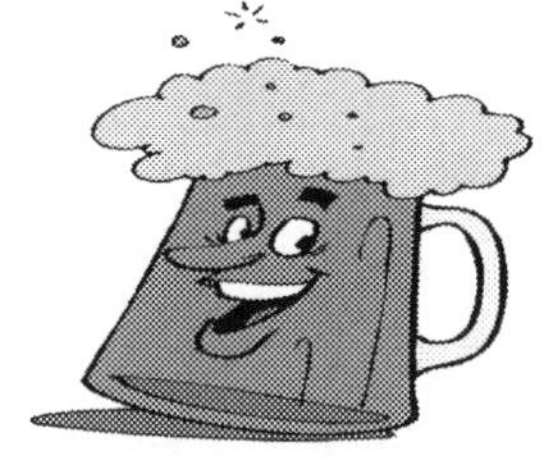

So add some variety by changing the foods you eat by experimenting with new flavors. This ensure you stick to eating healthy. Also remember to choose the most nutritional rich foods you can from each food group each day. Those packed with vitamins, minerals, fiber and other nutrients but lower in calories. Pick foods like fruits, vegetables, whole grains and fat-free or low fat milk etc. Get the most nutrition out of your calories. You could use up the entire amount on a few high-calorie items, but chances are you will not get the full range of vitamins and nutrients your body needs to be healthy.

# Remember these tips:

Let us start with some simple quick preliminary eating tips.

- Emphasizes fruits, vegetables, whole grains, low-fat dairy.
- Go for variety in you diet. It will deliver more nutrients and make you feel more satisfied.
- Include lean meats, poultry, fish, beans, eggs, and nuts.
- Avoid saturated fats, trans-fats, cholesterol, salt and sugar.
- Eat fresh vegetables as much as you can.
- Add one or more new foods each week to your diet.
- Eat organically grown foods where available.
- Most packaged foods have a nutrition facts label.
- Use the % daily value (DV) column when possible 5% (DV) or less is low, 20% (DV) or more is high.
- Check servings and calories, look for serving size.
- Choose the most nutritionally rich foods you can.
- Exercise daily, children should have 60 minutes of activity daily.

**Hopefully this book will get you off to a great start and a healthier life and well-being!**

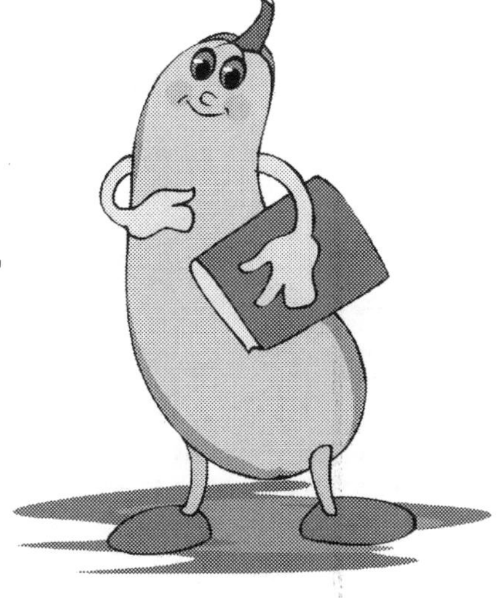

# Here is a tip to remember:

**If its white throw it out!**

White flour, white sugar, white salt, white bread, White paste, These foods are refined and have very little nutritional Value. Replace with whole grain products. For sweeteners use honey, rice syrup, barley syrup, white grape juice, pear juice. Try replacing salt with sea-salt, garlic power, onion power for seasoning.

# A sample of a nutritional breakfast

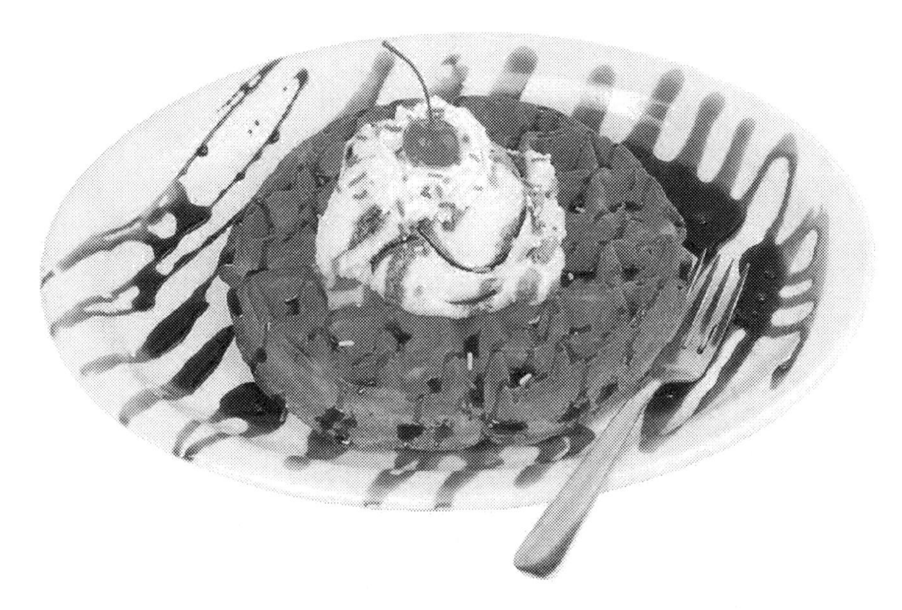

Remember breakfast is the most important meal of the day! So start you day with the right nutrients. Such as a nice whole grain waffle with blueberries, sliced peaches walnuts, and yogurt on top. With a grass of fruit juice. This will boost your thinking power, boost your vitality. There are countless other benefits, would be impossible to go through them all. But the message is, healthy food choices can make you look and feel great. Also you can try a bowl of whole grain cereal with some berries, and a couple of slices of whole grain toast, and fruit juice. And maybe a nice cup of coffee or tea.

## Sample of a nutritional lunch

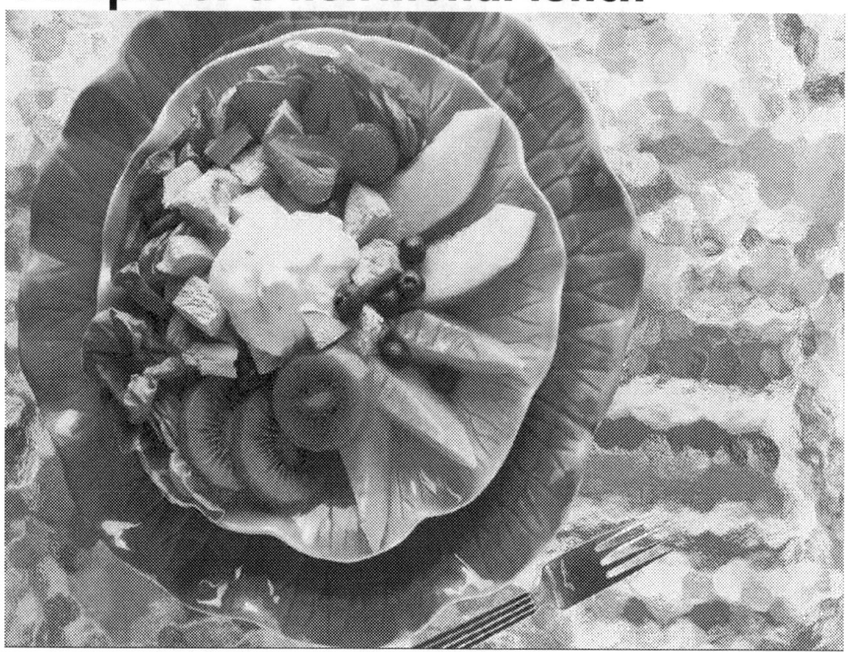

Pictured above is a good example of a great balanced lunch, a salad, with sliced kiwi, sliced cantaloupe, sliced honey dew, strawberries, blueberries, chopped chicken, on a bed of lettuce and spinach with some low-fat yogurt.

## Sample of a nutritional dinner

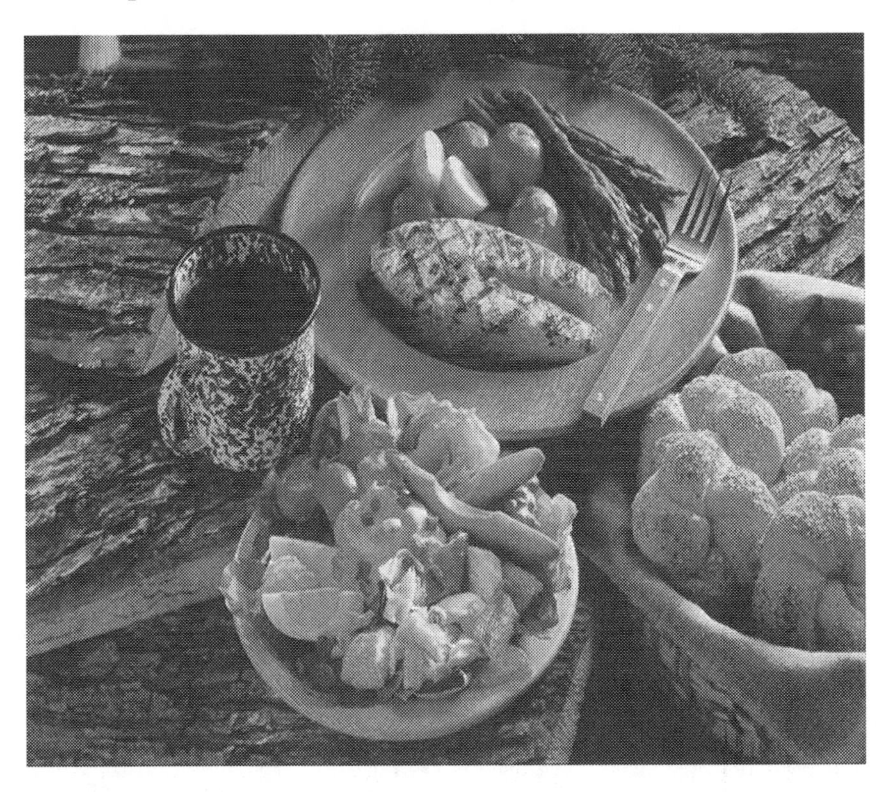

Pictured above is a good example of a balanced dinner with all the food groups, fish, steamed new potatoes, steamed asparagus, whole grain bread, and a nice salad consisting of boil egg, cantaloupe slices, mushrooms, artichoke, cherry tomatoes on a bed of spinach with a lemon, olive oil, cider vinegar dressing, and some green tea.

# A Final Note About Natural Foods

How you prepare and eat your food also affects the way the body and brain uses it. Over-cooking some starches can be similar to pre-digesting them, thus causing them to feed their sugars into the blood too quickly. Also over-cooking will eliminate a lot of the nutrition from the food such as vitamins, minerals, etc. Eating sugary food after a meal of legumes for example, may slow the absorption of sugar and prevent the sugar blues. The rate at which sugar from food enters brain cells is measured by the glycemic index (GI). Foods with high glycemic index stimulate the pancreas to secrete a lot of insulin, which starts the roller coaster. Foods with a low glycemic index do not push the pancreas to secrete much insulin, so blood sugar levels are steadier.

Proteins affect brain performance because the provide amino acids, from which neurotransmitters are made. Neurotransmitters carry signals form one brain cell to another. The better you feed these messengers, the more efficiently they deliver.

Putting the right food in helps, but it is important to get it out as well. That is why I nominate fiber as the unsung body food hero. There are studies that show people eating a good fiber diet had their mind clearing up once their system was cleaned out. Fiber helps detox the body. The body stores foreign substances and toxins in fatty deposits. So, in many cases, people may be carrying up to ten or more extra pounds of unhealthy toxic waste. And people wonder why they are so tired, have digestive disorders, headaches, joint pains, constipation and poor memory just some of the toxic disorders from eating an unhealthy diet.

The way people breathe can have a dramatic effect on your health, oxygen is a powerful detoxifies. Deep breathing is the key. Most people breathe in a shallow manner, thus depriving the cells, organs and glands much needed oxygen. Oxygen literally feeds the blood and cells, as it detoxifies the organs and glands, and is just as important as adequate supplies of water and good natural food.

In studies, children scored higher on test when on a regimen of daily foods full of the nutritional benefits such as vitamins and minerals etc.

Remember if you are on a blood sugar roller-coaster, with sugar highs and sugar lows. The ups and downs of blood sugar and adrenal hormones can also stimulate neurotransmitter imbalance, causing you to feel fidgety, irritable, inattentive and even sleepy. This is not the most conducive state for efficient brain function. It is equally important, however, to recognize the foods that diminish brain power. Alcohol and some drugs just kill brain cells directly, but there are many less obvious brain attacking foods. Artery clogging foods can lead to restricted blood flow to the brain, and high-glycemic-index foods cause terrible blood sugar swings that make both your body and your mind irritable and sluggish.

**These are a few bad brain foods:**
Alcohol, artificial food colorings, artificial sweeteners, colas, corn syrup, frostings, high-sugar drinks, hydrogenated fats, nicotine. As mentioned, alcohol just goes in and starts killing brain cells. Nicotine causes constriction of capillaries, which restricts blood flow to the brain, which reduces the delivery of good things like glucose and oxygen. Hydrogenated fats are more subtle, causing heart disease and general clogging of the arteries that eventually results in the same effects long term as the short term effect of nicotine. Since all three of these can kill you in addition to hurting your brain, you may want to replace them with healthy foods and drink.

**Stop Smoking and live a healthy life!**

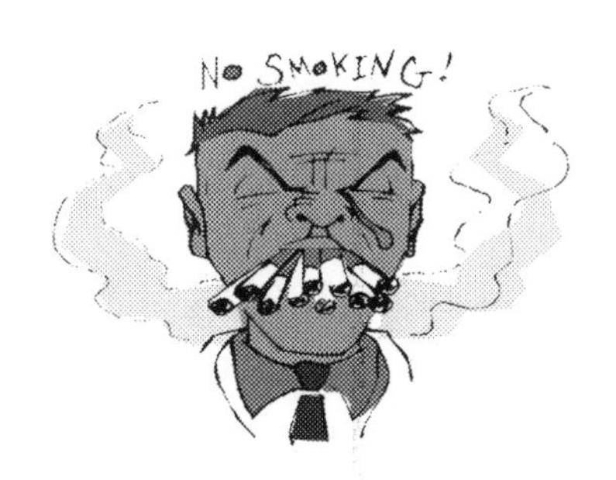

Here are some high protein, low carbohydrate, high tyrosine foods that are likely to rev up the brain are seafood, lean meat, eggs, soy and low-fat dairy products. High carbohydrate, low protein, high tryptophan foods that are likely to calm the brain include beans, legumes, nuts and seeds such as almonds, sunflower seeds and sesame seeds.

From here it just gets complicated. People respond differently to differing ratios of protein to carbohydrates in meals, there are also subtle sensitivities (not quite allergies) to foods that vary from person to person. Experimentation is called for, and since it is your body, you have to do it yourself.

# Index

# Index

# NOTES

# NOTES

**Hopefully this book has got you off to a good start for a long and healthy life**

*If you look at what you do not have in life, you don't have anything. If you look at what you have in life, you have everything!*